IF
SYMPTOMS
STILL
PERSIST

IF SYMPTOMS **STILL** PERSIST

Theodore Dalrymple

Illustrations by Nick Newman

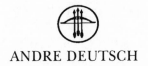

ANDRE DEUTSCH

The following articles all appeared in *The Spectator*
in 1994 and 1995

First published in 1996 by
André Deutsch Limited
106 Great Russell Street
London WC1B 3LJ

CIP data for this title is available
from the British Library

ISBN 0 233 99012 7

Printed in Great Britain by
WBC, Bridgend

Foreword

It is two years since the first collection of *If Symptoms Persist* was published, and the symptoms have definitely persisted. This is hardly surprising: traits such as the widespread British aversion to civilisation are not to be changed (if at all) in the twinkling of an eye, or by government fiat.

Much hope is placed in certain circles in a change of government, surely soon to occur. But, as the Romanian proverb has it, a change of government is the joy of fools. How any sensible person who has had even a brief encounter with British officialdom, at any rank in any department, can repose his hopes for national regeneration in a change of government is to me totally inexplicable.

However, I am not implying that all the changes which have taken place in the last fifty or a hundred years have been for the worse. There never was a golden age when criticism of the *status quo* would have been misguided. In my own father's lifetime, for example, life expectancy in Britain increased by 50 per cent and the infant mortality rate declined by more than 90 per cent. One would have to be an obscurantist indeed not to recognise that behind these figures lies a staggering transformation in the lives of untold millions.

And yet there is a pervasive and unshakeable feeling that the material betterment which has undoubtedly taken place has not conduced to human happiness as it ought to have done, or in the way which well-meaning social reformers anticipated. Remove hunger and hardship, it was supposed, free men from material anxieties, and Man would finally become fully Human.

The result has not been altogether encouraging, at least in Britain. I write these words during a short trip to Argentina, a country with a much more tormented and tumultuous recent history than Britain's. Yet in two thousand miles of journeying through Argentina, I have not seen in the faces of the people there that deliberate rejection of and hatred for civilisation which may be seen on British faces within a few hundred yards of every Briton's front door.

Of course, I know Britain much better than I know Argentina. To listen to ten thousand patients is a better way to get to know a country than to hire a car and travel the same number of kilometres through it. If I were a doctor working in the slums of Buenos Aires or Rosario, no doubt I should also come to the gloomiest of conclusions about Argentina.

Yet the Argentinians do not tattoo themselves like savages as the British do; nor do they wear that sullen expression of vacant aggressiveness, in search of a *casus belli* against the world, that so appals foreign visitors to our shores. The problem with the British is not that they live in an unjust society; it is that they think they do. Knowing nothing of history, nothing of geography, nothing of philosophy, they have no standard of comparison except with an impossible ideal (or daydream) relayed to them by television, advertisement, glossy magazine and film. They thus come to the conclusion that they are the most downtrodden and wretched people on earth. And, in thinking so, thus they very nearly succeed in becoming.

1

In the eternal struggle between doctor and patient, I told a medical student last week, the patient always has the upper hand. This is because, while the doctor is constrained by a code of behaviour, the patient is not: he can use any means he likes to bring about his desired end.

These profound reflections were occasioned by a patient who had not worked for many years and evinced a grim determination never to do so again, as long as he lived. The medical student had asked, as I signed yet another sick note testifying to the patient's supposed illness, how one distinguishes inability to work from unwillingness to do so – a good question. The distinction, I replied, can only be made in the case of the self-employed, when it is obvious. In conditions of social security, unwillingness and inability shade imperceptibly into one another. If I refused to sign the sick note, the patient would almost certainly do something which would indisputably make him sick. A doctor has to learn to accept blackmail, I said, with a good grace.

'They tell me I should pull myself together,' the patient had said. 'But I'm not a pair of curtains.'

This 'thing', which pressed down on him, he said, like a heavy rock, had started early in his life. He was a nervous child, and even now he was afraid of dogs.

'Every time I see a dog, I remember the dog what bit me in the bum when I was six,' he said, 'and I start to tremble.'

He was a delicate in those days, too.

'I was never allowed to box like the other kids because of trouble in the earholes. They said it would make it worse.'

Being of small stature, he was easy prey, and had

1

remained so ever since.

'I was even bullied by one of my best friends, he did it crafty, like. He would come up to me when no one was looking and thump me.'

In later life, his relations with his wife had taken a turn for the worse, and he had resorted to an overdose.

'I took some tablets what the doctor had give me, and he's never got over it. When I came out of hospital and I went to see him, he had me like a lion in a cage. He was walking round the surgery. "You took all them tablets," he said, "and I'm never going to prescribe no more tablets for you." And he never has.'

No one had ever liked the patient.

'But I like company,' he said. 'I'm only human.'

Even when he tried to find out how and why a neighbour or a relative had died – 'friendly, like' – no one would tell him anything.

'People die, and they won't tell me nothing. The body-snatchers, I call it.'

His wife had proved that he had been effectively doomed from the day of his birth.

'How?' I asked.

'She's interested in numerology. She's got a proper book about it by a bloke called Count Cheerio. She's added the numbers of my birthday, and it comes out to an unlucky number, just like I bet yours comes out to a lucky one. It's scientific: numerology's a proper science, like astrology.'

'And medicine,' I murmured.

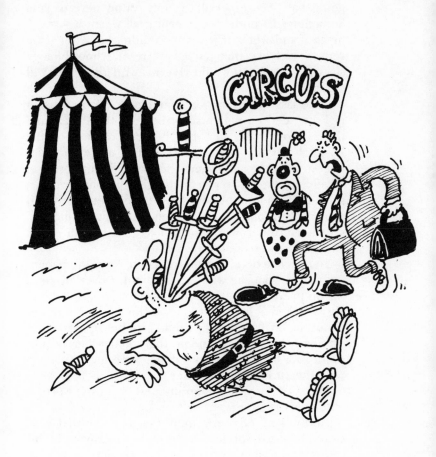

'Oh God he's taken an overdose!'

2

The course of true love never did run smooth, but the going has been especially rough round here of late. Sometimes I wonder whether it is all worth it – sex, I mean – and whether it really wouldn't be better if we reproduced like that old favourite of school biology classes, the *hydra*. It would save an awful lot of time and trouble.

Take last Thursday, for example. A young Muslim girl attended outpatients not because there was anything wrong with her, but because coming to the hospital was the only way she could make an assignation with the boyfriend she was not supposed to have. Each time we try to discharge her from the clinic, she begs us not to: but on this occasion her family had grown suspicious of her frequent attendance, and had sent her brother, who looked like an ayatollah of the Rushdie fatwa school, with her.

In order to deceive him, we had to keep the patient – if that is what she was – in a room for over an hour, for on previous occasions her visits to the hospital had always taken at least that long. If the family found out about the boyfriend, they would lock her up, force her on to a plane to Pakistan and there marry her at gunpoint to a brutal villager – if she were lucky. If not - well, then it might be murder.

I'm sure the young man in question wasn't worth it – he never is.

And talking of young men, that very Thursday an example of the species was brought to casualty by his step-grandmother, who had found him trying to electrocute himself in the bath. Earlier in the day, she had found him trying to plug himself into the light socket, and had decided enough was enough. Over to the medical profession.

He was dressed in those baggy jeans fashionable among joy-riders and young burglars; and his face bore the mark of Cain, namely the Indian-ink tattooed blue spot on the cheek, which proclaimed him a graduate of what used to be called Borstal.

He could see no point in continuing his existence (I am paraphrasing) because his 14-year-old girlfriend had thrown him over. Not only did she not wish to see him, she wished *not* to see him.

'Why is that?' I asked, smelling a rat.

'When I'm out of my head, I hit her.'

Further questioning elicited the fact that he was as frequently out of as in his head, and that only the week before she had attended hospital with a broken cheekbone.

'Can't you phone her, doctor, and tell her how much I love her?'

Clearly, there was romance in the air that day, because a couple of hours later a man appeared with gashes in his left wrist. He had done it because his fiancée had thrown her engagement ring at him. They had had a quarrel at a bus-stop, and he had head-butted her. Apparently, her dress was ruined by the blood from her nose.

'I can see her point of view,' I said, as mildly as I could.

'But it was only a one-off, doctor. I told her I'd never do it again, I love her too much for that.'

3

The origins of science are lost in antiquity. Some argue that the forerunners of today's Nobel prize-winners were Mesopotamian necromancers; of this theory I am not qualified to speak. Suffice it to say that all of us in our daily lives put forward hypotheses which are falsifiable by observation – the very touchstone of science, according to the late Sir Karl Popper. Yes, we are all scientists in our own way.

Take, for example, the lady whom I saw last week who had developed a theory which was entirely falsifiable. She had given birth to her fourth child about five months previously.

'I was really proud, doctor,' she said, 'because I'd gone through pregnancy all on my own, without a man.'

She wasn't claiming virgin birth, of course; only that she had booted out the paternal parent of her forthcoming offspring as soon as she learnt that she was pregnant again.

He was the father of all her children, and she had ended her affair with him because he was very violent towards her. He had punched and strangled her in what I now know to be the usual marital fashion, and had tried to abort her first two children by kicking her in the stomach. After her common-law divorce, she had thrown herself and her children upon the cold mercy of the state.

'I hope you don't mind me asking,' I said, 'but why did you have four children by such a man?'

'You don't understand, do you, doctor?'

'No, I'm afraid I don't. I'm trying, but I still don't.'

'I loved him. He wasn't like that all the time.'

'Could a man be like that all the time?' I asked. 'Even the worst imaginable?'

'No, I suppose not.'

'After all, even Frederick West wasn't killing people all the time.'

'No, doctor.'

'Was he violent towards you straight away?'

'No, not straight away. Only after we started to live together.'

'But before you had your first child?'

'Yes.'

'But you still had children with him?'

'I thought he would change.'

And that was her grand hypothesis, refuted a thousand times since. Hypothesise in haste, falsify at leisure.

My next patient, as it happened, had discovered relativity theory. He had taken rat poison because of what he called the pressures. The week before he had slashed his wrists. Next time, he said, it would be hanging – though he wanted to leave hospital as soon as possible because United were playing at home that evening.

'What pressures?' I asked.

'I lost my job last week.'

'Why?' I asked.

'Time-keeping.'

'You mean, not time-keeping?'

'Well, yeah. Then there's my wife.'

'What's wrong?'

'She's about to drop.'

'Drop what?'

'Drop a baby.'

'Drop a baby?'

'Give birth, like. And we've already got two nippers.'

He had pub-crawler's nose – somewhat out of true – and a scar on his forehead. I suspected that the police might be adding to the pressures.

'Yeah, I got a case next week.'

'What is it?'

7

'ABH. I might go down.'

'What happened?'

'Well, this geezer was mouthing off and I got pissed off with him so I hit him. They say I broke his nose, but it wasn't me, it was the pavement.'

The pavement came up to meet his nose in the same proportion as his nose went down to meet the pavement: that's relativity theory for you.

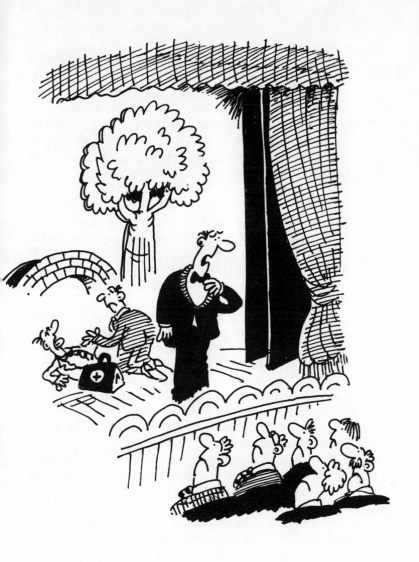

'Is there an administrator in the house?'

4

It is by reflection on the small phenomena of the universe that we are led insensibly to the profoundest truths. That is why the study of trivia is not itself trivial. Consider the following question: why is it that when people say of themselves that they are easily led, they are always talking about drug-taking or burglary and never about art appreciation or the study of higher mathematics?

The question takes us straight to the innermost depths of the human heart. No one claims to be easily led to what is good for him, but only to what is bad. Some might argue that this is because only the bad is deemed to require an explanation, the good being self-explanatory, but such an answer could only be given by those fortunate enough to have had little contact with the human race.

No, the fact is that Man – especially the young of the species – flies to the bad like iron filings to a magnet. I see instances of this natural attraction every day.

A 13-year-old girl appeared in casualty last week complaining that there was a tape recorder and radio transmitter in her stomach. It is true that she had a remarkable amount of ironware inserted in her body: I have never seen so many rings in one ear or metal studs in the nostril of a nose.

The trouble with 13-year-olds nowadays is that they have been so well-fed that they are as big as adults; and a rebellious child's mind in an adult's body is a terrible thing.

She replied to all my questions by alternately sulking and pouting. This gave me an idea: perhaps instead of beauty contests, which are no longer socially acceptable, there could be sulking and pouting competitions. My patient would have stood a good chance of honours in such a contest. Extracting answers from her was like getting Mr Gromyko to say yes.

I persisted, however. I used the method which has secured me small victories over bureaucracies the world over: I adopted a manner which finally persuaded her that it would be less trouble to answer me than not.

The tape recorder in her stomach was no ordinary tape recorder: it recorded her thoughts and played them back to her out loud. This was both frightening and boring.

The tape recorder lodged in her stomach was due to the ecstasy she took every weekend in one of the local clubs which are the El Dorados of impoverished young imaginations. She recovered completely after a couple of days in bed and small doses of tranquillisers.

I spoke to her again. She came from a completely normal background: she didn't know who her father was, she had two stepfathers whom she hated, the second of them only eight years older than her. Her mother was also young enough to be her sister, and they argued constantly over the time she should be in – not later than midnight, according to her martinet of a mother.

'Why do you take the ecstasy if it makes you feel so awful?' I asked.

'I want to stay up all night. All the uvvers take it. I'm easily led, I suppose.'

I tested her reading ability: she could pronounce some of the words, but had no idea of their meanings. You can lead a girl to drugs, but you can't make her learn.

5

Doctors are not immortal, and – less surprising still – neither are their relatives. And thus I found myself last week on the way to London, to visit an aged uncle of mine who had been taken ill and admitted into one of the great teaching hospitals there.

The train was full, and I was glad to get a seat – but not for long. The young lady next to whom I sat gave off the sound and smell of modern British culture: the tish-tish noise of what I suppose I must call a personal stereo, which resulted in a certain rhythmic titubation of her head, combined with the stench of a cheap hamburger, which she consumed with agonising slowness. Surely, if passive smoking is bad for one, the passive consumption of junk food must be even worse. Can one be passively cholesterolled, I wonder? Here is something worthwhile for the Department of Health to spend millions of our money studying.

Still, I was prepared to give my fellow-passenger the benefit of the doubt, as she was reading a *Teach Yourself* book, while she destroyed her hearing and clogged up her arteries. We none of us start out perfect, and self-improvement is an admirable thing. I myself have used several *Teach Yourself* books in ephemeral attempts to learn the languages of countries I proposed to visit for a week or two. Then I noticed what it was that she was teaching herself: *Successful Gambling*.

I looked over her shoulder and caught a glimpse of a chapter summary:

Do not stake more than you can afford to lose.

I turned to look out of the window. Fortunately it was dark: most of Britain looks so much better in the dark, when you can't actually see it.

We reached London: too many people, mostly badly dressed, with vile expressions on their faces. Then I noticed a poster which offered a cheap excursion fare to Preston, and I felt reconciled to London: I should have thought any fare to Preston, however low, was extortionate.

The hospital was one of those horrible modern buildings done on the cheap. The only thing that could be said in its favour was that it was better than Addenbrookes, in Cambridge, with its giant crematorium chimney next to the entrance, *pour encourager les autres*, I suppose. I don't know anyone who goes to Addenbrookes without immediately thinking of Auschwitz.

And then Addenbrookes has its wonderful system of levels, rather than floors, designed – I daresay – to prevent the Wehrmacht from ever finding the paediatric wards, there to commit its characteristic atrocities. You wouldn't have guessed that the hospital was built a quarter of a century after the conclusion of hostilities. Altogether a typical triumph of British architecture.

Well, I found the ward to which my uncle had been taken. I wanted to announce myself to the staff before approaching him, but this was easier said than done, for it took me five to ten minutes to find a member of staff to announce myself to.

And when I found her, she was a bird of passage: a pleasant and well-meaning Australian nurse working a shift for an agency, to fund the next stage of her Grand Tour around the world.

Age could not wither her, but for reasons rather different from those adumbrated by Enobarbus: out of her rather skimpy blue uniform emerged legs in black knitted leggings, and a green, American military-style T-shirt was clearly visible above the *décolletage* of the same blue uniform. It remains only to add that something resembling vegetable soup had clearly been strained through much of her uniform, though at some time in the past, since it had now dried.

I point no finger, I blame no one. I am a camera. I must therefore record that the ward was clean and pleasantly spacious. My uncle, a respiratory case, is approaching 90 years of age. He had slipped down the pillows and I said it would be better if he sat up. There was no one to help me to help him to do so.

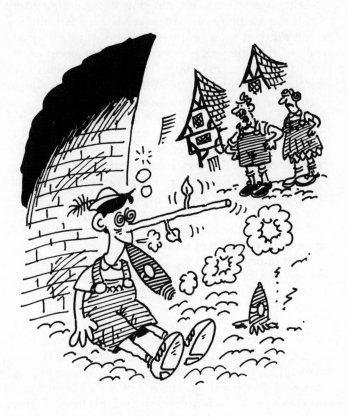

'Pinocchio's a typical product of a one-parent family.'

6

I was sitting in my office during a hiatus between out-patient clinics last week, thinking in a desultory way about the Meaning of Existence. Alas, try as I might I could think of none, but perhaps this was because my train of thought was interrupted by the sound of the ward television drivelling through the walls. An astrologer was reading Mr Blair's horoscope: Saturn was in the ascendant, the Moon was somewhere else entirely, it was all very exciting and unusual, and meant that . . .

I rushed out and turned the television off. It seemed to me likely that the man in the bed nearest it, who had complained of invisible gerbils gnawing constantly at his legs, would not be much interested in Mr Blair's starry destiny. After all, when you are pursued by rodents, even the highest marginal rate of income tax must seem a matter of slight importance.

Most of my patients would agree in any case that life has no meaning. And even those who once thought otherwise are soon brought to the same conclusion.

An Indian shopkeeper consulted me because of a host of symptoms, which affected every part of his body – he even had a burning sensation in his hair.

He had migrated to this country a third of a century ago and had worked hard in a factory to save enough money to buy his shop. His ambition had been to put his children through university, and this he had done; and then he wanted to leave them a tidy sum, to ease their passage through life. But in the last few years he had been held up so many times in his shop at knife-point that he had sold it to the first bidder – to whom he passed the martyr's crown. The fact is that the shop-keepers in our area have as much chance of escaping unscathed as the early Christians in the arena.

The police had been most sympathetic and kind to him, of course, but had caught none of the culprits and had told him that in any case there were plenty more where those came from.

My patient woke up every night sweating; his heart pounded in his chest. His entire view of the world had changed, and now every stranger was an armed robber until proven otherwise. He had devoted his whole life to his business, and had not had the time to develop other interests; and now even the local park was closed to him since he was mugged there. It is a truth universally acknowledged that a small man in a suit and a tie is asking to be robbed.

'When I came to this country, it was very nice,' he said. 'They delivered to your door, and no one was taking. Now it is a rubbish country.'

Anyway, back in my room I stopped contemplating the meaning of life, and turned my attention to a somewhat smaller, but more clearly defined question: why did I no longer have a wastepaper basket under my desk? Pilfering, perhaps? A management economy measure?

The ward smoke alarm went off in the midst of my reflections. I went to see what was happening: the alarm was being tested. It took three men to test it, one up a ladder, one with a clipboard at the base of the ladder, and one – a Fire Prevention Engineer – to oversee operations.

And then, suddenly, the whole meaning of life became clear to me: so to arrange things that we survive until tomorrow.

7

How odd the human race is, and getting odder by the hour. One might have supposed, for example, that the life of the British underclass is so deeply unattractive in all its aspects – financial, gastronomic, sartorial, musical, etc. – that almost every sentient being would do everything in its power to avoid such a miserable existence. On the contrary: an increasing number of the children of Indian immigrants strive to join the back-to-front-baseball-hat-shaved-head-multiple-nose-ring-fuck-you culture, which is surely more primitive than anything seen on the Indian sub-continent since the extinction of the dinosaurs.

An Indian girl came to our hospital last week who had forsaken her education at the age of 14 for the joys of drinking in the local park. She soon expanded the range of her interests to include clubs, pubs, drugs and brawls. Her parents then tried to marry her to a respectable boy, but the family of her intended groom learnt of her habits, and called it off. When her family discovered that her younger sister was also going astray, they blamed her and threw her out of the house.

She fell at once into the clutches of a young black man, who tried to supplement his Income Support by a little light pimping. When she resisted him, he beat her; she slashed her wrists and was sewn up in the hospital.

What she needed, of course, was a strong, stable, loving relationship. On the ward, as it happens, there was just the man for her: he was on what is known as 'the sick' because of his drinking. And he had just swallowed bleach because he and his wife had broken up. Was there ever a better sign of true love and devotion?

'Why did you separate?' I asked.

'We had our ups and downs, like everybody else.'

'And what did the downs consist of?'

'The usual.'

'Any violence involved?'

'Not what you'd call violence, no.'

'What *would* you call it, then?'

'Well, I smacked her about a bit. Not all the time, like.'

'Did she ever have to go to hospital?' I asked.

'Good God, no,' he replied – perish the thought. 'Only the once.'

'What happened then?'

'Well, I thought she'd been talking to this bloke in the pub. I'm not normally violent, but I wanted to rip his fucking head off. I broke his nose and a few ribs. I wish I hadn't done it now. Anyway, I got hold of my wife and took her home after.'

'And then what happened?'

'Well, we was arguing, and I said she fancied him and she said she didn't, and I don't know what happened, I just grabbed her with my temper.'

'With your temper?'

'Yes, I admit I got a temper on me. I'm not violent any other time, though.'

'And she left you after that?'

'Yes. She called the police in and said she was afraid of me. I said if she was afraid of me, how come she's stayed with me for eleven years? But the Bill said I had to go, and I ain't seen her since, nor none of the children.'

'How many?'

'Seven.'

Yes, altogether a perfect match: he free of any encumbrances, she – the Indian girl striking out for freedom – searching for someone a little older and more experienced to guide her through life's small

19

difficulties. I wondered whether such a match could be arranged, but on second thoughts I realised there was no need. As I left the ward, I noticed that they had already found each other.

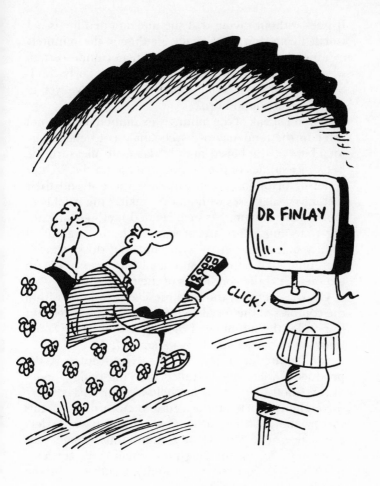

'We're losing him'

8

It goes without saying that the unexamined life is not worth living; but then again, neither is the minutely examined one. In actual fact, I am not quite certain what kind of life *is* worth living, but I am fairly confident that, if such a life exists at all, I have yet to encounter it round here.

When I speak of the minutely examined life I do not refer to the tendency of psychoanalysis to encourage members of the bored middle classes to measure the petty vicissitudes of their emotional life on the Richter scale; or of philosophers to polish without end their metaphysical glasses without ever taking the trouble to look through them. No such refined methods of wasting time and effort are practised within a radius of twenty miles of where I write; but that doesn't mean that only philosophers and analysands examine in tedious detail the conditions of their existence.

On the contrary, those whose lives are lived within the compass of the social security system are no less apt to ponder the minutiae of their quotidian being. I am thinking in particular of my patient, Mr X.

Mr X attends a Day Centre. This centre is the product of what may be called the Ping-pong Theory of the Good Life, which has held sway in this country throughout much of the century. According to this theory, the good life, at least where the lower orders are concerned, consists of a minimum income plus unlimited access to ping-pong tables in concrete bunkers – designated Community Centres – in the middle of vast housing estates.

One might have supposed that anyone caught up in this dreary world would at least have displayed solidarity with his fellow-unfortunates; but not a bit of it. Anyone who supposed such a thing would have shown himself profoundly ignorant of the true ghastliness of human nature.

Mr X is at present exercised to the point of obsession about a new rule which has just been decreed – God knows by whom, it is one of the characteristics of this world that one can never discover who is responsible for what – that henceforth only women will receive free haircuts, whereas it had been the custom from time immemorial, or at least from 1978, that men too could have their hair cut there free of charge.

Mr X, I hasten to add, has nothing against women; no, not even against his own wife.

'After all,' he said, explaining her negative reaction to the latest government budget which had left her £2.50 per week better off, 'she's got to pay for her cigarettes, so £2.50's not a lot.'

It was the principle of the free haircut for women but not for men which upset him.

'It's discriminatative,' he said, the outrage increasing the mobility in his mouth of his false teeth.

He went on to describe further instances of injustice at the Day Centre.

'Not that I'm a tell-taler,' he said. 'But this chap just went to the toilet for a wet, so he didn't bother to pull the chain, but he was told off and given a warning if he did it again he'd be out on his ear. But this woman I know didn't even wash her hands after a mess, never mind just a wet.' He assured me that the story was true, because he had heard it 'by mouth of word'.

He also assured me that he was not a misogynist in general.

'A woman,' he said, 'may give her body for sex, but on the other hand, doctor, she could be kind to children or animals.'

9

Is Man a machine? Philosophers have argued over this for centuries, as philosophers will (it is their job, after all), but I have arrived at my own conclusion, which is the following: alas, no, Man is not a machine.

Machines – at least these days – are so much more polite than Man. They always say (or print) please and thank you, which is quite unlike Man. For example, the other day I was at a cash-dispensing machine, of the kind at which an alarmingly high proportion of my patients have been mugged by Man after withdrawing their cash, and as it counted out my money it asked me most obsequiously to wait. When finally it asked me please to take my money, I found myself saying 'Thank you' in reply.

Compare this civilised exchange with what was written in the medical notes of the first patient on one of my ward rounds last week. 'Only history available from patient,' the exhausted junior doctor had recorded: ' "Fuck off!" '

Whenever I hear a young person saying that he or she would like to work with people, therefore, I feel like exclaiming, 'Don't waste your time, devote yourself to machines, at least they'll be grateful!'

The patient in question eventually came round, of course, and no longer confined himself to bisyllabic answers. But it emerged that his ill-mannered replies to the junior doctor's questions were not entirely co-incidental. As the ancient Romans said, *In lysergic acid diethylamide veritas*.

He was quite unrepentant. One might have supposed he had been kidnapped and brought to hospital against his will, instead of having been deposited in the emergency department like a sack of coals by his so-called friends. I wouldn't be surprised if he tried to sue us for assault.

In the course of our conversation, I asked whether he had ever been in trouble with the police.

'Yeah,' he said. 'But nothing serious.'

'What, for example?'

'Fighting.'

'In what circumstances?'

'Football matches. You've been to football matches, haven't you? You know what it's all about?'

'No, what is it all about?'

'Well, you watch the game and then you have a bit of a fight, like.'

Did he really think that I, a middle-aged doctor, spent my Saturday afternoons shouting for the Reds and then beating up those who had shouted for the Blues? I looked deep into his eyes: I think he did.

I soon discovered other instances of human discourtesy on the ward. A boy of 17 had cut his wrists because his parents had kicked him out and he had needed somewhere warm to stay for the night.

'Why did they kick you out?' I asked.

'I lost my job, and I couldn't pay my rent no more. They said if I couldn't pay my rent I'd have to go somewhere else.'

'And why did you lose your job?'

'The boss told me to make a phone call, and I told him he could shove his phone up his arse.'

Then there was the daily crop of beatings: for example, a young Pakistani bride beaten up on her wedding night to establish the principle that obedience is the best policy.

My pager went off and asked me to ring another hospital.

'Please hold the line while I connect you to the operator,' said the machine. 'We apologise for any delay, but will try to answer you as soon as possible.'

No, Man is definitely not a machine.

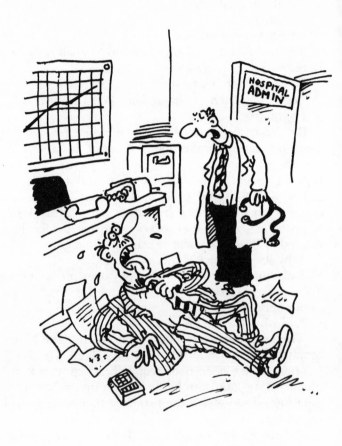

'I'm afraid you closed the Coronary Unit'

10

Compared with the depravity by which our hospital is surrounded, all other depravity – the licentiousness of Sodom and Gomorrah, the decadence of Weimar Germany, the concupiscence of Tiberius Caesar – is but the decorum of Tunbridge Wells.

I was moved to these comparisons by the non-appearance at work one morning last week of one of our ward doctors. She had been mugged the day before in the hospital car park, and was badly shaken. She had gone to her car and had noticed a couple of youths peacefully removing a radio from another vehicle.

Quick as a flash, they sized up the situation and, seeing that she was small and defenceless and carried a handbag and that there was no one around to witness anything that they might do, rushed over to her, threw her to the ground and grabbed her bag. They could finish off the radio job later.

This doctor has had a run of bad luck, as it happens. A couple of months ago, she turned the corner in a hospital corridor and slipped and fell on some vomitus recently deposited on the floor by a drunk. Apart from the sheer indignity of it and the repulsiveness of the experience, she had hurt her back and was badly bruised.

And a few months before that she had been attacked as she parked her car near a restaurant, where the staff from the ward were having a dinner. As she stopped her car by the kerb, a brick was thrown through the window, the door opened, and she was pulled out and thrown on to the ground, her necklace ripped off and her bag snatched.

She is a kindly, inoffensive person, and so it must have seemed to her as if the world had lost its natural order and was intent upon returning evil for good. Of course, there was no question of catching the culprits, or even of trying to do so.

Another of our doctors was robbed on her way to work last week: she pulled up in her car at some traffic lights, the passenger door was wrenched open and her handbag snatched. She managed to grab hold of it and a tussle ensued, which in the end she lost.

Not surprisingly, the ward staff sat in the office and discussed the problem of crime. Of the three nurses present, one had been mugged recently on the bus, and another's house had been burgled. She had left for work dressed, for once, in her uniform – normally she changed at the hospital. As luck had had it, there was a youth loitering outside her house, who saw her depart and made the most of the opportunity. Who says entrepreneurship does not flourish in England?

We all agreed that the situation – unlike the latest crime statistics – was not a joke. But what should be done about it? The ward sages agreed that there was no point in excessive leniency.

'We should be like Saudi,' said Sister. 'Just amputate their hands. They wouldn't do it again.'

'Waste of anaesthetic,' muttered another nurse.

'Who said anything about an anaesthetic?' asked Sister.

'Nurse, nurse!' The voice of an elderly patient penetrated into the ward office. 'Can I have a glass of water, please?'

'Yes, of course, dear,' said Sister. 'Just coming.'

11

There is a brand of insanity, or so it is alleged, which consists in this: that the sufferer, so-called, does not know the difference between right and wrong. This ignorance is not contingent, as would be (for example) an ignorance of the history of Paraguay, which, in theory at least, can be rectified. With the morally insane, as they used to be known before more neutral-sounding terminology was adopted, it is more like trying to teach the blind to see and the deaf to hear. And the sufferers actually do not suffer very much: it is the people around them who bear the burden of their malady.

But do such people as the morally insane actually exist? I am not sure: for my part, I have never known anyone who lacked the very concepts of right and wrong. On the other hand, those who do not know how to apply them are legion.

I am driven to these somewhat abstract reflections by the case of a nurse who worked on one of my wards and was recently mugged by two young men, who overpowered her easily. She was in a part of the city where artists and other undesirables congregate, and she had done some shopping. She stopped at a bank to withdraw a little money from its dispensing machine, and was then followed by the two young men.

As soon as she noticed them, she realised they were up to no good and crossed the road. They followed her and grabbed hold of her.

'Give us your money,' they demanded.

She said she had none.

'You're a liar,' they said. 'We saw you at the cash-point.' And then they hit her, blacking both her eyes.

It didn't take them long to make her dispense to them the £20 which the machine had just dispensed to her: not a large sum, perhaps, for the average mugger, but more than the average nurse can afford to lose.

'Next time,' said the muggers as they ran off, 'tell us the truth.'

What astonished the nurse – once the initial shock had worn off and after she had received treatment in her own hospital – was the moral outrage which the muggers appeared to feel when she told them an untruth. They believed that those whom they would call their 'clients' if the worked for Social Services had a moral duty to tell them the truth when asked a question. They wouldn't have hit the nurse if she hadn't lied, and therefore the nurse had asked for, and deserved, what she got. It was a form of punishment for telling lies.

Let us now imagine that, *per impossibile*, the two muggers are caught by the police. Let us also imagine that they undergo interrogation and that, because the police know that they are not being told the truth, the two suspected muggers are given a good beating – still *per impossibile*, of course.

Eventually the two men confess to the mugging and sign confessions. The magistrate then sentences them to community service because, before this unfortunate incident, there is no record of them having been other than fine, upstanding citizens.

Is the moral that the two young men draw from their experience that they should always tell the truth to the police? Or is it that the 'system' is evil, that the world is against them, that so-called respectable people are liars, and that all their morality is hypocrisy?

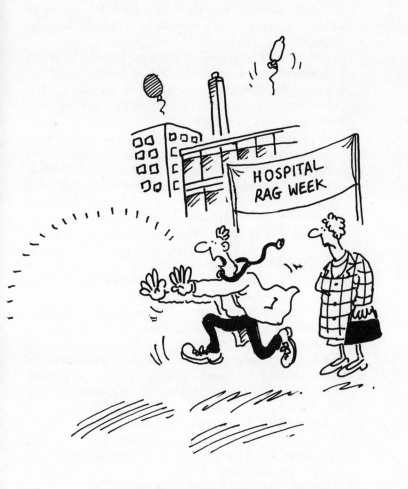

'We're raising money for some beds'

12

I am entirely in favour of British fathers paying for the upkeep of their children. Someone has to pay for the little bastards (I speak both literally and metaphorically), and I can't see why it should be me, the taxpayer.

The trouble is that when the Government invents a bureaucracy such as the Child Support Agency to enforce retrospectively an otherwise excellent principle, things are bound to go wrong and the principle itself to fall into disrepute.

A patient of mine, whose wife had walked out on him a couple of years ago, tried to hang himself after receiving a letter from the CSA demanding £5,000 in arrears of maintenance. Payment was to be made within fourteen days. Furthermore, he was told that he was henceforth to pay £250 a month to the agency. The worst of it was that only a fraction of this money, decided upon unilaterally by the CSA, would actually be paid to his wife and children.

Since his net pay per month was slightly less than £800, these sums seemed excessive in any case. He had saved some money, about £1,000, to give to his ex-wife, he already paid for his children's clothes and holidays, and was about to come to an amicable agreement with her concerning regular maintenance. However, the law no longer recognises such agreements where one of the parties draws some kind of social security benefit.

He tried for two days to telephone the agency, but received only a recorded message in reply that all lines were busy. Then he went to the offices of the agency, but was not admitted. Being a man of limited imagination, he then tried to hang himself.

I called the agency on his behalf. Of course, I did

not use the number distributed to the public, but found another number direct to the local head-quarters. I got through to a voice which I recognised at once, from experience, as being that of a British bureaucratic zombie, for whom work is a painful interruption of entertainment.

'How are you spelling that?' she asked, when I gave my patient's name. Since his name was as straightforward as Jones, I could only conclude that this was a delaying tactic and that she hoped I was in a public call-box and that my coins would run out before she was actually required to do anything. She also asked that I spell the words of his address, although each of them was equally straightforward.

'I'll try to put you through to the right office,' she said at last.

I was put through to another British bureaucratic zombie. I repeated my patient's name and address, and had to spell them once again. I explained that he had tried to hang himself. His case was called up on the computer.

'Yes, he owes £5,000,' said the bureaucrat.

'That's rather a large sum for someone who earns £800 a month,' I said. 'It's most unlikely he would have it.'

'We don't expect him to pay it all at once.'

'Your letter says within fourteen days.'

'But it says that if he has any problems he should phone.'

'He tried for two days but couldn't get through.'

'We're very busy here.'

'He tried to speak in person to someone in the office.'

'The public's not admitted.'

'I think when you write such letters, you should make it clear that you do not expect payment immediately, in a lump sum.'

33

'Yes, we've had a lot of feedback like that.'

A phrase started repeating itself in my head, like a tune you can't get rid of: government of morons, by morons, for morons.

'I think I should write to your superior, asking that your letters be more tactfully phrased,' I said. 'What is your superior's title?'

'The Customer Services Manager.'

That afternoon, I had a clinic in the prison. How long, I wonder, before prison governors are called Customer Services Managers? In many documents prisoners are already called *clients*.

13

There's nobody quite like a patient for grasping the wrong end of any stick which is proffered him. Ever since the Government decided of its own accord to insinuate the so-called Patient's Charter through every letterbox in the land, patients have been getting above themselves. They imagine they are imbued with all manner of rights, and now attend hospital in a state of anticipatory grievance.

A man who thinks he has many rights knows neither gratitude nor contentment. If they are fulfilled – well, they are his rights. He has received only his due, and there is nothing to be grateful for. But, if they are unfulfilled, he conceives himself ill-used and goes into a sulk.

On Friday last, my gloomiest prognostications concerning the dangers of giving the English the impression that they had rights were utterly vindicated. Two patients turned up at my clinic, the first an hour and a half, and the second two hours, late.

'You've got to see me within a quarter of an hour of my arrival,' said the first. 'It's in the Patient's Charter.'

I have nothing but contempt for this fatuous document, the paltry attempt of politicians to deflect discontent from themselves, but even it does not say anything so silly.

'You are supposed to be seen within half an hour of your *appointment*,' I replied majestically, but, alas, this was a distinction too subtle for his understanding.

The second late-comer was even wider of the mark.

'You've got to see me now,' he said, 'because I missed my last appointment.'

A third patient wanted a prescription for which I thought there was no medical indication. I should perhaps explain that I am in favour of people being allowed to purchase whatever medication they choose, but that does not mean I should have to prescribe whatever they choose.

The patient left in a cloud of expletives, and fifteen minutes later I received a phone call from the local law centre whither he had repaired at once. The lawyer said he wanted to discuss his client's prescription with me.

I said he didn't have one, so there wasn't anything to discuss. I put the phone down most emphatically.

But it isn't only in the invention of rights that the English now show ingenuity: it is also in the committal of wrongs.

That same day, a patient aged 75 described to me how her sister had met an Australian during the war, married him and gone to live in Australia afterwards. She decided last year to visit her for the first time in nearly half a century, and went to her building society to draw out £1,500 to pay for an air ticket.

Alas, on the way to the travel agent someone managed to rifle her bag without her knowledge, and when she arrived at the agent's, the money was gone.

'The police told me that the thieves used a powerful magnet to draw back the zip. They said it was a lot of money, but I was lucky they didn't hurt me.'

'I hope it wasn't all the money you had,' I said.

'Oh no,' she replied. 'I've still got an emergency fund: enough to pay for my funeral, like.'

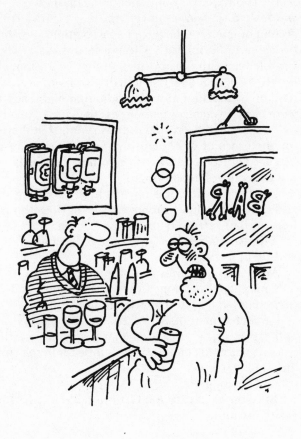

'I drink, therefore I can't remember who I am.'

14

The morning before my clinic in the prison last week, I was woken at three o'clock by the irruption into my dreams of the sound of my next-door neighbour's car alarm. By the time I reached my window to survey the scene, two masked young men had smashed one of its windows and had removed the car's radio, to the accompaniment of the owner's impotent cries from his bedroom of 'Stop that!' The police were later able to console him with the information that he was not alone in his loss: this was the fourth car from which the dynamic duo had removed a radio that night, and they were clearly tracing a path across the city.

A certain tiredness, and the awareness that there but for the grace of God went my car, left me more than usually ill-disposed towards common criminals – *aka* my patients – the following day.

The first of them was one of those snivelling drug-addicts who would rather break into a thousand homes than refrain from taking heroin.

'They've charged me with breaking and entering, and theft,' he said.

'Are you going guilty or not guilty?' I asked.

'Guilty on breaking and entering, not guilty on theft. They can't pin that one on me.'

He and a mate had broken into someone's house and taken a table. Realising that it was not worth the wood it was made of, they had dumped it in the garden and done a runner.

'So I'm not guilty.'

'But you would have taken the table if it had been worth anything?'

'Yeah, of course.'

As it happened, his mate was to be my next patient.

'He's got a worse rabbit than me,' said my first

38

patient cryptically.

A worse rabbit? Did they breed these generally inoffensive creatures in their spare time, I wondered? But how nasty could rabbits be? Suddenly, his true meaning dawned on me: a worse habit.

Enter the young man with the worse rabbit. He was 20 years old and told me that he stole only to feed his rabbit. Generally – this case being an exception – he stole only from countesses and duchesses, like.

'They can afford it,' he said.

'That's hardly the point,' I said.

'They must be able to. If they can afford to have a chair worth £15,000, they can't miss it, can they?'

'Have you asked them?'

'No, of course not.'

'Then you're hardly in a position to say, are you?'

'They get their insurance,' he said.

'And where do you suppose the insurance money comes from?' I asked.

'I don't know,' he replied.

'People like me, who pay premiums,' I said.

'But I wouldn't steal from people like you.'

Another point in his favour, he said, was that he would take things only from the ground floor, thus avoiding giving the countesses and duchesses an unpleasant fright in their bedrooms.

So successful had he been as a burglar of antiques that he had been able not only to feed his rabbit with the proceeds, but to buy antiques of his own with which to furnish the flat where his devoted girlfriend lived with him.

'How long do you think you'll be sent down for this time?' I asked.

'Well, the judge'll probably say I'm a professional.'

Up till now he had been only a juvenile.

'But you are a professional,' I said.

'I suppose I am,' he conceded. 'That means I'll get

39

a three or a four.'

'Well, then, your girlfriend's going to bugger off with your antiques, isn't she?'

His face dropped.

'She better not,' he said.

'Why not? You can afford it.'

'I'll break her fucking legs.'

15

There was a crisis in the ward last weekend. Two patients who had previously evinced a desire to die by their own hand by taking an overdose were caught, *in flagrante delicto*, in that life-enhancing and (in the absence of appropriate precautions) life-creating activity which is popularly known as sexual intercourse. This would not have mattered so much had they chosen the linen cupboard as the venue for their assignation rather than the staff toilet. This small space is to the staff what the Temple of the Tooth is to Ceylonese Buddhists; and if you knew our patients, you'd also know why.

The hospital carpenters were called at once and an extra lock installed. The miscreants had been apprehended because, so pressing had been their desire (once, that is, they had discovered that after all they weren't going to die), that they omitted to lock the door from the inside. Now one needs a key to get inside in the first place.

One of the disgraced patients was an alcoholic, known to me of old, who assumes in the face of a figure of authority a whipped-dog expression which brings out the worst in me.

'Why did you take your overdose?' I asked him.

'They gave me some pills in the pub,' he replied.

'And did you have to take them?' I asked, my voice like a drill.

The possibility of refusing to do so had not previously occurred to him. He remained silent.

'Do you suppose,' I continued, 'that if someone were to come into my room and give me a handful of pills that I should take them?'

'But you're a doctor,' he replied.

Obviously he believed that I belonged to a

completely different and superior order of beings. I confess that the thought crossed my mind as well. If Aristotle were alive today, his natural slaves would be natural overdosers.

We turned to the question of alcohol. It wasn't long since he'd been dried out in the same hospital bed as he occupied now. In the course of his last admission, he had seen carnivorous bats flying towards him, which he had tried to escape by running naked round the ward. He had returned to drinking immediately on discharge from hospital.

'You see, I'm surrounded by alcohol, doctor,' he said in a tone which implied there was a vast conspiracy outside hospital to prevent his sobriety.

'So am I,' I said.

'But it's completely different for you, you're not an alcoholic.'

'Now let's get this straight,' I said. 'You're an alcoholic because you're surrounded by drink; whereas I'm not surrounded by drink because I'm not an alcoholic.'

'That's right,' he said.

It was time for him to leave hospital, but he didn't want to go.

'You've got to stop me drinking first, doctor,' he said.

'How? By sending you to the Arabian desert?'

No; by finding out why he drank in the first place.

'Let's start with something simpler to answer. Why didn't you keep your last out-patient appointment?'

'I couldn't. I had something to sort out with a woman.'

'And you couldn't have spared a couple of hours from the sorting-out to come to hospital? Or two minutes to phone to let us know you weren't coming?'

'No. I'm telling you, doctor, if I hadn't gone to sort things out with her, there would've been chaos, absolute chaos. You see, she's having my baby.'

'And what's happened now?'

'Oh, we've split up. She don't want to see me no more, never again.'

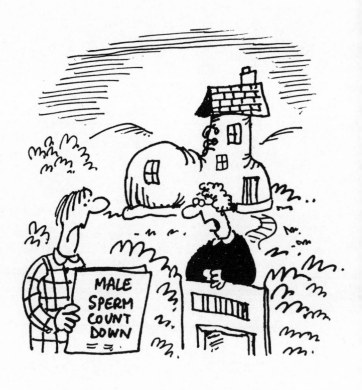

'I've got no children and I don't know what to do.'

16

The entire nation has been plunged into deep, indeed inconsolable, mourning over the untimely demise of Frederick West. News of his death came as a shock, to me as to others, and naturally I began to ponder the big questions, as philosophers call them, such as whatever happened to Smith, to whom I was called out some time ago while I was on duty for the prison, who had eaten an entire fluorescent light tube in his cell, glass, metal, attachments and all?

It was lucky for Smith, I thought, that he was not in the ex-Soviet Union: there, in the good old days, he would have been charged with stealing socialist property.

I asked him why he'd done it. He was trying to kill himself, he said, before the prison food, which he thought was poisoned, could do so.

I phoned the surgeon at the nearest hospital.

'I've heard the food in there isn't very good,' he said. There was much joking in the casualty department about light snacks.

It isn't only about prison suicide that the Government is concerned, of course. We doctors have been given the responsibility by the Department of Health of reducing the numbers of suicides in the nation as a whole by 15 per cent by the year 2000.

The way to achieve our goal is through the coroners' courts, of course. Some time ago a wealthy and successful man I knew swallowed 200 tablets and a bottle of rum. The coroner asked me whether I thought he might have taken them by accident.

I was about to answer with a ringing and confident no, when the coroner made himself a little clearer: was there even a one in a million chance he had taken them by accident?

'Er, well, I suppose so,' I replied.

The coroner (and the man's family) relaxed, an open verdict was returned, the family was £750,000 the richer and an insurance company the poorer by an equivalent sum, at least until it put my premiums up.

But to return to suicide in prison. I'm not sure whether Judge Tumim's well-intentioned proposal that people at risk of suicide in jail should be placed under continuous observation would decrease the suicide rate there, but I think it would have a sizeable effect on the unemployment rate, given the frequency with which prisoners mention the possibility of doing away with themselves. Those who don't want to go on Rule 43 (which segregates them from the rest of the prisoners), but who – often quite understandably – don't want to go to the rest of the prison either, use the threat of suicide as a means to remain in the hospital wing.

Come to think of it, an elementary prerequisite of justice is that everyone should be treated alike. As we know, at least 100,000 people a year take overdoses in this country, and within a year 1,000 of them will have killed themselves: surely they – the 100,000 – deserve no less than continuous observation, or are we to conclude that they are second-class citizens by comparison with prisoners?

For continuous observation to be even minimally effective, two people at a time must carry it out: one is not sufficient. Since there would have to be three shifts of eight hours each, six observers per overdoser would have to be found, plus a further four to cover weekends, sickness and holidays. A million people would be thus employed. Truly, it is an ill wind which blows nobody any good.

17

Multiculturalism, someone once remarked, is not cous-cous: it is the stoning of adulterers. Of course, there is more to it than that, as I hope soon to demonstrate. But the problem which really interests me is not multi-culturalism, but what may justly be called *aculturalism*. It seems to be the triumph of our technological age to have raised a generation with no discernible culture whatever.

I am aware, of course, that this has been the com-plaint of middle-aged men since the time of Plato, if not earlier: it just so happens, however, that this time, as I myself enter middle age, it is true. How else can I interpret the inability of four-fifths of the 17-year-olds I come across to name three writers?

So if people have more than one culture, this repre-sents a great advance, as far as I am concerned, on hav-ing none at all. Many of the minorities are rather good at absorbing British culture, better, in fact, than many of the natives. The problem with multiculturalism, in my experience, lies elsewhere.

I don't recall among the scores of my Indian patients a single one driven to despair by white racism, though they all know that it exists. On the other hand, there are many who bear the scars – in some cases quite literally – of the communal conflicts of the subcontinent.

Last week, for example, a young man of 17 fled to the hospital to escape his persecutors. The majority of people who do this are mad, pursued as they think they are by the CIA, the Mafia, the KGB or MI5, but he was not: his life was truly in danger.

He was a Sikh, but a non-observing one who cut his hair and his beard. At school he had become friendly, in an innocent and platonic way (he assured me), with

47

a Muslim girl. They were seen talking together on a few occasions by that great instrument of oppression and bigotry, the community. Some time later, the Muslim girl fled her home because her family were plotting a marriage and a life of domestic drudgery for her, to which she could not reconcile herself. The Sikh did not know her whereabouts.

Her family, ever mindful of their reputation in the community, sought a scapegoat on whom to blame her departure, and alighted on the Sikh.

'They hate us and we hate them,' said my patient, explaining the relations between Muslims and Sikhs.

One day, as he was walking along the street, four of the girl's relatives jumped on him, held him down and slashed his face with a knife. He needed plastic surgery afterwards.

The police caught his assailants, but this was not the end of the matter. The community had approved so strongly of the action in defence of their family's honour taken by the four men that it had given warning that further attacks on the young Sikh were to be expected. The laws of the land were as nothing compared with the laws of honour: and it was well worth spending a lifetime in jail to avenge the terrible wrong of a Sikh boy talking in public to a Muslim girl.

The boy left the city, but his parents still live in fear.

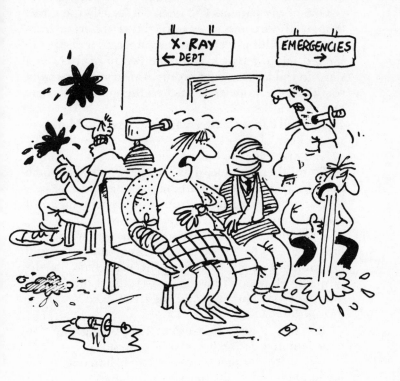

'Sod it — we're missing "Casualty"'

18

Sometimes I feel I should like to become a hermit in the desert, to avoid all contact with humans. Even the honey and locusts might be an improvement on National Health Service sandwiches. Oh for a cave in which to contemplate the meaning of existence, instead of having to answer my radio-pager every four minutes and speak to relatives and teach students!

One of my patients last week felt exactly the same, though his circumstances were rather different from mine, as was his preferred means of escaping them. He wanted me to admit him for the rest of his days to a ward in the local lunatic asylum, through whose twilit corridors the hopelessly mad shuffle and gesticulate their lives away.

'But you can look after yourself,' I said to him.

'No I can't.'

'You know how to boil an egg at least.'

'So do them people. They don't just sit and watch the telly, you know, they do the washing-up as well.'

'But why on earth do you want to join them?' I asked.

'They don't have no responsibilities or worries in life. I'd like to be one of them. I'd swap the house and everything I've got for life in the main block of the hospital. They don't have to worry about the gas bill and the pipes bursting, and the stairs need repairing terrible.'

'But you've got to have something wrong with you to be admitted to the hospital,' I protested.

'I suffer from convulsions and bad habits, doctor. It's my mother's fault, she never taught me to stick up for myself properly. And I suffer terrible from earache – it's in the family, earache is.'

'Earache is in the family,' I repeated feebly.

'Yes. And another thing: I've got a black spot in my eye. I've had it ever since I was born. You don't think it could be serious, do you?'

'No, not if you've had it all your life.'

'I used to watch it go up and down the wall like a creepy-crawly. I was fascinated by it. I didn't pay no attention to lessons at school because of it. I just used to watch it all the time and the teacher wouldn't believe me when I told her what I was doing.'

'But a black spot in your eye is not a reason to spend the rest of your life in a lunatic asylum.'

'I've had nerves all my life, doctor. They wouldn't take me in the army because of them. They examined me and said my nerves was like violin strings, and I could only go in the army in an emergency.'

'But that was many years ago.'

'I'm still nervous, doctor. I do things what I can't control. For instance, I've had several affairs. The last one was worse than the others because she had a house and a car. And I had to have treatment to cure me of her.'

I told him that, nevertheless, I thought a lifetime in the asylum was excessive in his case, and that perhaps another outpatient appointment would do.

He reached the door of my room, and then turned to me.

'There are three types of men who get stuck on an island, doctor. There's them that make the best of it, there's them that try to escape, and there's them that give up. I'm one of them.'

To which island did he refer? Surely not to Great Britain?

19

I am not by any means an Islamic scholar, and therefore cannot comment on what the verses in the Koran
with regard to the treatment of women *really* mean: but
I suspect that many Muslim men choose to interpret
them in a way similar to that in which the late Robert
Maxwell interpreted the duties of a trustee of a pension fund.

That, at any rate, is how it seems to me. Last week,
two Muslim women were admitted to our ward having
taken overdoses, the only way known to them of leaving their homes. Both had been married by arrange-
ment in Pakistan, but their subsequent fates differed
slightly.

The husband of the first had deserted her four
months after the wedding, leaving her pregnant. She
returned to England, where she fell in love with a man
who was willing to accept her child as his own.
Unfortunately, her husband arrived from Pakistan four
years later and demanded his conjugal rights, backed up
by a threat of suicide from her mother if she did not
return to the errant husband.

She did return to him, he accused her of being a
prostitute and he beat her accordingly. Several times
she had attended the accident and emergency department of our hospital with cuts, bruises and dis-
locations; demurely, she lifted her scarf and showed me
a bruise on her neck, where her husband had punched
her a few days before.

She was not allowed out of the house for a moment
without an escort of one of her brothers, and even then
very infrequently. Her present imprisonment at home
contrasted with her period of freedom during her husband's desertion of her and her cohabitation with her
lover: and now she wanted to die.

I suggested divorce instead. But how, she asked, could she divorce her husband? Her letters were opened at home, and she was not allowed to use the telephone. I planned a cloak and dagger operation: she would come with her child as an outpatient to the hospital, where we would have a lawyer and a social worker waiting for them, and they would spirit her and her daughter away, perhaps to another city, while her ever-jealous and suspicious husband waited for her to emerge from the consultation. I would face his wrath alone.

As for the second patient, she had always wanted to be a lawyer, but her father had allowed her to go to school only one week in three (sufficient to keep the school inspectorate quiet, but not enough to take exams).

At the age of 17, she was married off to a man who wished to marry her as little as she wished to marry him. They returned from Pakistan to England, where they insisted on divorce, much to the disgust of her father, who believed that because of it the family name was ruined for ever.

'You're lucky we haven't killed you – yet,' said her father.

He'll wait to take her back to Pakistan, of course, before killing her. During the month she was there for her wedding, a 16-year-old girl in the same village was caught talking to a boy. Her father killed her with a meat cleaver and threw her body off the roof of his house to make it look like an accident. My patient remembered the blood in the dusty street. The father was arrested briefly, but released thanks to public opinion and a bribe.

My patient awaited her murder, if not quite with equanimity, at least with dignity. She realised her over-dose had been foolish.

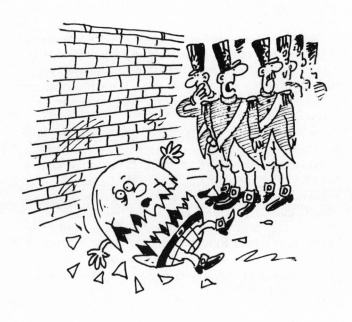

'You're in luck — here comes Princess Diana.'

20

When I walked on to the ward one morning last week I surmised from the exhalations of stale alcohol which greeted me that I might have to endure an insult or two before the end of the day. One of the worst things about being a doctor is that you have to pretend that repulsively bad manners are a sign of suffering.

The insult wasn't long in coming. I approached the first bed, which contained a patient who, just before his arrival in hospital, had smashed up his common-law wife's flat.

'Good morning,' I said.

'Piss off, will you,' he replied, looking at me with such concentrated malevolence that even I, who am no stranger to the ways of human malice, was taken aback.

I recovered a little, and carefully wrote in the notes 'Piss off, will you,' so that whenever he attended our hospital in future, he could be assured of a frosty, hard-hearted reception.

'How are you feeling?' I continued, turning the other cheek.

'I'm telling you to piss off.'

The patient in the next bed was a truly terrifying specimen, a young man with bulging muscles and receding forehead, with 'Made in Britain' tattooed round his left nipple. This was a redundant piece of information, for on his biceps were tattooed unfurled Union flags, guarded by bulldogs, their snarls revealing rows of fangs. The man's head was shaved, the bristly scalp punctuated with white scars from wounds inflicted by bottles, crowbars, etc.

He had been admitted to the hospital unconscious. Apparently, he had bought some methadone (the drug used in the treatment of opiate addiction) in a pub and swallowed rather too much of it.

'How much did it cost?' I asked him.

'Five quid.'

'Why did you buy it?'

'How the fuck should I know? I was drunk, wasn't I?'

I changed the subject. I had noticed a large scar across his neck.

'How did you get that?' I asked.

'I cut my froat.'

'Why?'

'I don't know. I had enough, I suppose.'

So had I. Truly I had glimpsed the abyss, the abyss of modern life. Poverty is not quite the word for it, conjuring up as it does images of children without food or shoes. Indeed, I thought my patient looked unhealthily healthy.

In the afternoon, I had an outpatient clinic. To raise money, the hospital management has now installed televisions in the waiting area, on which local services are advertised, including those of a faith healer who has succeeded (he says rather pointedly, considering the location) where many have failed. The waiting patients watch the screen as a rabbit watches a stoat.

My first patient was a man whom I remembered as having been exceptionally truculent during his last appointment. My recollection proved correct: for my note about him on that occasion read 'Fuck off' and nothing else.

I was relieved to discover that today he was in a better mood. He had thought over his truculence, and had asked for another appointment.

He leant over my desk and looked at his notes, which were open upon it.

'I never said that,' he said.

'Yes, you did,' I replied.

'No I never. I said, "Fuckin' 'ell".'

'All right, then,' I said, and I crossed out 'Fuck off'. Pursing my lips, I replaced it carefully with 'Fuckin' 'ell'. By all means let us be accurate.

21

A patient came to me in a state of some agitation last week because Her Indoors (his name for his wife) had just left him, for no apparent reason.

'Were you ever violent towards her?' I asked.

'No,' he replied virtuously. 'I've never even given her a smack in the face.'

Then was he ever violent towards anyone else? I asked only because the word *hate* was tattooed in Indian ink on the knuckles of his right hand.

'I don't go looking for trouble, if that's what you mean, but if trouble comes to me I know how to look after myself, like.'

And when was the last time it had been necessary to look after himself?

'A week ago. This bloke was eyeballing me in the pub, so I hit him.'

'And what happened then?'

'They had to take his teeth out and put his skull back together.'

I saw from his past medical notes that he had taken several overdoses. Had he thought of doing so again because of his wife's desertion?

'Oh no,' he said. 'I've committed suicide three times, I wouldn't want to commit suicide again.'

My next patient suffered from cold feet, both literally and metaphorically. He told me that he had hypothermia, especially of his extremities.

'Would you like to see my feet, doctor?'

'Not really,' I replied – he was not altogether clean, and I could already smell his feet in my mind's nose.

Too late! His shoes and socks were off, and he was pointing eagerly to the parts which often went numb with cold. 'Rat poison works by hypothermia,' he said, putting his socks back on. 'Did you know that? I've often thought of taking rat poison. I think it would work with me.'

'Why haven't you?' I asked.

'Because I might come back as a worm or a fly,' he replied. 'Do you believe in reincarnation, doctor?'

'Not really.'

'You believe that when we die, that's it, then?'

I feel uneasy to discuss religious or philosophical matters with my patients, so I remained silent.

'What do you think about abduction by aliens?'

'To tell you the truth, I don't give it a lot of thought.'

'They say that over a thousand people have been abducted by aliens.'

'I have my doubts.'

'Oh well.' He prepared to go. 'Can you recommend anything other than rat poison to kill me, doctor? Something painless.'

'I'm afraid not.'

'Pity. When can I come to see you again, then?'

I walked into the ward after he had gone. There were three attempted suicides in a row. The daughter of the first had accused him of raping her. ('I swear on the Holy Bible, doctor, I didn't do it, it's her mother what put her up to it, she wants me out of the house.') The second took tablets in a police cell after he was arrested for having used his car as an offensive weapon, by driving it to squash an acquaintance who owed him £10 against a wall.

The third had slit open his stomach with a razor blade for the seventh time. ('I've just had enough, doctor, so why don't you go away and let me die?')

If only I could go away! Oh for an alien to abduct me to a higher, better, purer planet!

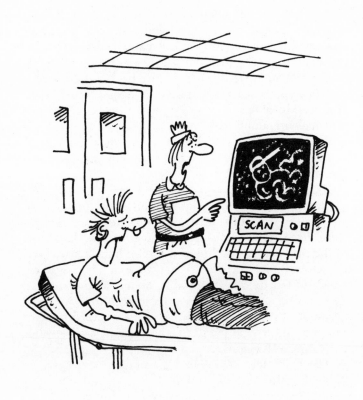

'Oh no — his baseball cap's facing the wrong way!'

22

Last weekend in the prison, a rapist was bitten on the chest by a murderer during a fight: a pity, I hear the feminists murmur, that the latter didn't have rabies. Personally, I was filled with admiration for the murderer's teeth, which somehow managed to get a purchase on the rapist's chest despite its complete absence of flesh.

There are fashions in prison fights, as in everything else. Not long ago it was for the ballpoint pen in the eye, but just now (thank goodness) it seems to be for the good old dependable, low-tech human bite. One of the prison officers was bitten on the same day by a prisoner suspected of harbouring cannabis in his mattress, who objected to the intrusive nature of the search carried out of his cell. Later, when he had calmed down a little, he ascribed his attempted mastication of the officer's finger to 'a misunderstanding'.

My first and only patient on the Saturday sick parade limped into my office. He had the scar of an old knife wound on his face.

'It's my knee, doctor' he said. 'I've had it for seven years.'

'I should think you've had it a lot longer than that,' I remarked.

'I mean the joint's loose,' he said, by way of clarification. 'I've been promised an operation in four months' time. But I've got pain all the time.'

'I'll give you a painkiller, then,' I said.

'I've got all this pain and you want to give me a painkiller?' he said, his facial scar turning livid with rage.

'Seems logical to me,' I said.

'Fuckin' 'ell. I want to see a proper doctor.'

'Are you saying that I'm not a proper doctor?'

'Yes.'

He had a point, of course. A proper doctor would have refused to have anything further to do with him.

Next day, though, he had become a little more reasonable and I agreed to see him again. The pain in his knee had evidently convinced him that painkillers might not be such a bad idea after all.

'What about this operation, then?' he asked, after I had written up his prescription. 'They keep promising it to me, and then they don't do it.'

'Why's that?' I asked.

'Because I keep coming in here. Every time they're going to operate, I get arrested and put inside.'

'You could try making this your last sentence,' I said.

'No, I couldn't,' he said firmly. 'It's my way of life.'

How many prisoners there are for whom prison is not home from home, but home *tout court*! The previous day I had met a vagrant alcoholic whose drinking had got too much even for him, and so he committed an act of criminal damage for once. I remarked on how pathetic his case was to an officer.

'Do you remember J—, sir?' he asked.

'Yes. A Geordie with a ferret tattooed round his navel.'

'That's him, sir. Well, he was released last week, and he was so upset he came back next day and smashed the glass door at the entrance. He's back in now.'

No, there's no place like home.

23

Last week I went up to a young patient in the ward who was sobbing quietly to herself in her bed, and asked her what was wrong. She had taken too many tablets in an attempt to kill herself, but had been caught in the act by her sister who just happened to be popping in at the time.

And why, I asked, had she wanted to kill herself?

She had had a row with her boyfriend, with whom she had lived for four years, ever since she was 15½ years old. He was nineteen years her senior, a divorcee, who accused her constantly of having an affair with another man. However much she denied it, he would not believe her.

This was a story all too familiar to me. It soon became clear that he was one of those insanely jealous men who allow their wives or lovers no freedom, who see evidence of their infidelity everywhere, and who consider everyone their rival. Such men are dangerous. 'Have you ever read *Othello*?' I asked.

'What's that?' she replied.

'A play by Shakespeare.'

'I'm not interested in Shakespeare.'

'A pity. Has your boyfriend ever hit you?'

'Yes, but not very hard. He's smashed up the flat a few times, though. And he says that if he finds out who I'm seeing, he'll kill him. But I'm not seeing nobody.'

'All the same, one day he could be very dangerous to you. And he's never going to change. After all, he's been like this ever since you've known him, and I'm sure he was like it with his former wife.'

'But he's never really injured me.'

'You can only be murdered once.'

'Most of the time he's very nice.'

'Murder doesn't take long.'

'I've been all right so far.'

'If I understand you correctly, you'd like to stay with him, but you want him to stop being jealous?'

'Yes, that's right.'

She knew in her heart that this was about as likely as that fish would sing. She was thus destined for years of pointless suffering. In the 1940s there was a Soviet defector called Kravchenko who wrote a book entitled *I Chose Freedom*; her autobiography, on the other hand, would be entitled *I Chose Misery*.

In the next bed was a 16-year-old girl whose boyfriend, aged 30, had visited her the previous evening. He approached her bed, moved her bed table to clear the trajectory of his arm, and punched her hard on the face, several times. He had an audience: two doctors and two nurses. Having completed his assault, he hurriedly left the ward, while the doctors and nurses asked the patient whether she wished to have her boyfriend prosecuted. She said no, and that was the end of the matter.

When I heard about it the following morning, however, I felt it should not be allowed to rest there. The impression had been given, and no doubt received, that our patients could be assaulted with impunity. I called our legal department to find out whether it was really true that prosecution in such cases depended upon the willingness of the assaulted parties to press charges. I described what the boyfriend had done.

'Why did he do it?' asked the legal department. 'Perhaps he had a good reason.'

'And what,' I asked, 'would constitute a good reason for a man to hit a patient while she is in bed, or indeed at any other time?'

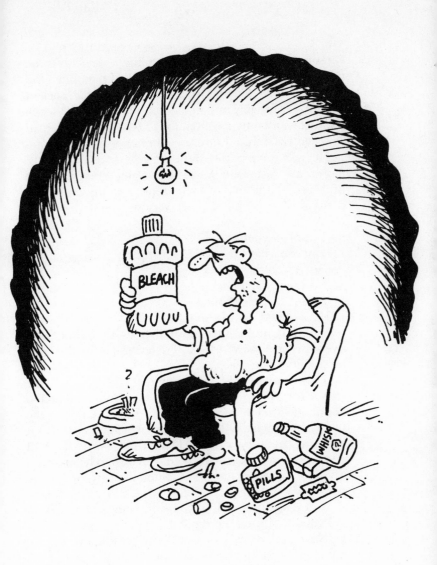

'I can't swallow this — it's past its sell-by date!'

24

I hesitate to pen anything resembling a cliché, but the trouble with children these days really is that they have no discipline. The irrefutable truth of this ancient lament was forcibly impressed upon me last week when I was consulted by a woman of 22 who brought her 3-year-old child into the room with her.

He was quite a nice little boy, or so I thought: a handsome face with lively, enquiring eyes. Alas, he grew bored after about half a minute in my room and demanded from his mother various objects from my table.

'I want the pen.'

'You can't have it,' said his mother.

'But I want it.'

'Well, you can't have it.'

'I want the telephone.'

He reached up to the table and a disaster (for the telephone) would have ensued had his mother not swept his arm away. A look of determination hardened on the little one's face.

'Fuck you,' he said to his mother.

Nature abhors a vacuum, and man abhors anarchy: law of one kind or another must prevail, even if it is the law of the jungle. This was the law which had prevailed with my next patient, a 14-year-old boy who had emerged from his school the day before to be accosted by three youths a few years older than he who were previously unknown to him.

'You're coming with us to town,' they said.

'I don't want to,' he replied.

'Never mind,' said one of them, pulling out a large knife and putting it to his throat.

They frog-marched him on to a bus as if he were under arrest. As they approached town, the three youths told him that they would show him someone with a gold chain and he was to snatch it on their behalf. He had better do as he was told.

However, when they alighted from the bus he managed to run off, and they did not catch him. They knew him now, though, and might return for him: last night he had nightmares.

That afternoon I went to the prison. I was waiting for the arrival of patients in my room when I heard two officers walk by.

'Suicides are not the best way to start the week,' said one to the other.

Before long an officer entered my room and asked whether he could 'put B— before me'. B— had been assaulted at lunchtime.

B— turned out to be a short man, rather plump, and was trembling with terror. He had a black eye, a split lip and sore ribs.

'What happened?' I asked.

'Three men burst into my cell,' he replied, his voice as unsteady as his nerves. 'Then they started punching and kicking me.'

'Why?'

'They thought I was a nonce. But I'm not: my cell-mate is, but he wasn't there. When they realised they'd got the wrong bloke, they said they was sorry, like.'

He was afraid to return to his cell, in case he were mistaken for a nonce by three more righteous burglars. But of course he wouldn't reveal who his attackers had been: to grass up is to break prison's first and most fundamental law.

25

Philosophers have long debated the moral justification of punishment – well, that's the kind of thing philosophers do, of course. But if they find it difficult to justify punishment in general, what would they make of prison in particular? If ever there were monuments to the vanity of human endeavour, prisons are they: except, unfortunately, that no society can quite dispense with them.

For a spectacle of sheer inspissated futility, it would be hard to surpass the daily intake into our penitentiaries of scores of minor wrongdoers who have failed, through cussedness or otherwise, to pay their fines. They are released after serving only a day or two, but in that short time much public money is expended, and the law made to look an utter ass. Is there really no one in these densely populated islands who can devise something better, or (which in the context amounts to the same thing) less expensive?

Last week, however, I did finally stumble upon a useful function which prison performs, other than keeping psychopaths under lock and key: I discovered prison as a means of contraception.

I interviewed two prisoners, one aged 22, a rapist, and the other aged 24, a grievous bodily harmer, who had between them 15 children, distributed between 11 different mothers (assuming no exact overlap in the objects of their inseminatory activities). Prison had brought a temporary end to their procreation, and could thus be considered as a kind of expensive prophylactic: one prisoner costing the taxpayer more to keep than a whole brood of such infants.

The two men regretted only that their children were able to see them infrequently, thanks to the expense of public transport, the meanness of social security payments and the reluctance of the mothers to visit the men who had deceived them. Otherwise they were happy enough: granted parole, they could expect to go forth and multiply again within a comparatively short time.

I try to be broadminded (it doesn't come naturally, I can assure you); I try not to sound like Mrs Grundy or Colonel Blimp. Yet, try as I may, I cannot imagine what, if anything, goes through the minds of the men and women who bring children into the world as insouciantly as I collected frog-spawn as a child or stole eggs from birds' nests. An African peasant desires many children to secure his old age; but why do the rapist and the GBH-er need so many offspring? Oh God! A beast, that wants discourse of reason, would pause longer before procreation.

Mind you, the two fathers weren't the only ones I couldn't understand that day. An absconder was put before me, a man who had failed to return from home leave to his open prison (where the regime was liberal, to say the least) and who, when he was recaptured, was brought to our more secure institution.

'Why did you abscond?' I asked.

'I didn't like open prison,' he replied.

'Why ever not?' I asked.

'Too much time on your hands.'

'Do you mean to say you prefer it here?'

'Yes. You don't have to think here.'

69

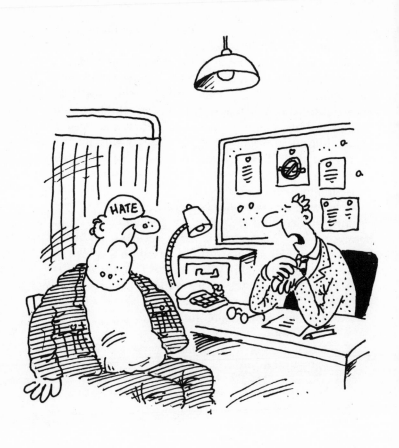

'I can tell you're angry — it's written all over your face.'

26

If it's lesser breeds without the law you want, you can't do better than Britain. The only law recognised in large parts of the country is the law of the biggest boot, the heaviest punch, the sharpest knife and the ugliest threat.

I noticed last week that one of my patients had a swollen and disfigured wrist. She had come about something quite different, but I asked her about her wrist nonetheless.

'My boyfriend done it,' she said.

'How?' I asked.

'During an argument.' She made a gesture as if she were breaking a twig: that was how he did it.

'What did you think?'

'I thought I mustah done something wrong to deserve it.'

I peered hard into her face: she was perfectly sincere. I asked her what conduct on her part could or would have justified her boyfriend's brutality. She was unable to say: her guilt was general and unattached to anything in particular which she had done.

'But I did tell the police,' she continued. 'I even pressed charges.'

'And what happened?'

'I dropped them.'

'Why?'

'He said if he was convicted, he'd lose his job, and then he threatened me. Well, not me exactly. He said he knew where my little boy went to school and he could easy get him.'

There was reason to believe that she was not the first woman whom he had treated in this fashion, but he had never suffered the consequences of his actions, except for the break-up of his relationships. He would bully his way through life like a knife going through polyunsaturated sunshine spread.

My patient had not been altogether wise in her choice of gentlemen friends. The one before the wrist-breaker had deserted her the moment she gave birth to his child, though apart from saddling her with this twenty-year liability, he was, she said, decent enough.

The man with whom she had taken up since the breaking of her wrist was, alas, a bounder. Large parts of his biography, as he related it to her, were blank, and suggested – to me at least – forced acceptance of Her Majesty's hospitality. He claimed to have amnesia for those lengthy gaps. Moreover, three weeks into their relationship, he began to see another woman. It was a purely platonic affair, he told her – and no doubt he told the other woman the same thing.

'But I want to believe him, doctor,' said my patient. 'I love him, you see.'

I got her half to admit that he was no good, but then she exclaimed, 'I need to have a man, doctor! Is that wrong?'

'No,' I said, admiring her will to love. 'But you need a decent man, a man who won't just exploit you.'

'But where do I get a decent man?'

Round here – impossible. A good man is above the price of cocaine. But it wasn't always like this: years ago, decent men were in the majority. I recalled a widow who said of her husband that he'd been 'golden'.

'He was a very good man, doctor. He never asked me for no sex, nor nothing like that, but when I was asleep, he'd help himself, like.'

27

I was on my way last week to the home of a patient –
or perhaps I should say to the home of an *alleged*
patient, for I had been called because he was lunging
drunkenly with a knife at his family, and these days,
such is the pervasive doctrine of the *Real Me* that the
doctor is called in such situations rather than the police
– when I noticed an eight-year-old boy performing
powerful and destructive karate kicks on a free-
standing street name. Naturally, I blame the council: if
they put up street names like that, what can you
expect? Equally naturally, I didn't stop to tell him to
cease his attacks on defenceless public property,
because he was in the company of his dad, who
appeared to take some pride in his precocious powers
of destruction, and might have been armed.

Fortunately, the consultation with the drunken
lunger was brief. His house was the only one for some
scores of yards with glass in the windows rather than
chipboard, and most of the cars in the vicinity were
held up by bricks rather than by wheels, properly so-
called. All the local grass was strewn with empty tins of
drinks, cigarette packets and polystyrene containers of
take-away meals; it came as no surprise that the members of his family (all female) were fat slatterns. By the
time I arrived, the patient had fallen asleep, emitting
Richter-scale snores, his head lolling upon bosoms of
which Jane Russell might have been proud. The bread
knife had escaped his grip, and lay upon the floor. His
family now denied that there was anything wrong and
were annoyed at my presence, which they had
requested only a few minutes before.

This was just as well, for I was late for the prison and
did not wish to be detained long. In the prison I was
consulted first by a type which every prison doctor will

recognise: the pony-tailed Buddhist.

The P-TB (for short) is always a vegan, because his principles not only do not permit him to eat the flesh of any animal, but consider the theft of eggs and milk from the poor suffering chickens and cows to be utterly reprehensible. The P-TB always speaks in a lowered voice, a kind of pious whisper, in case the unnecessary decibels should disturb the flies. The P-TB believes that even inanimate objects are suffused with a living spirit, and must therefore be respected.

It comes as a surprise, therefore, to learn that the P-TB is invariably in prison for armed robbery or GBH. Do not his principles apply, then, to the owners of small shops, bank clerks, etc.? Apparently not, for the P-TB is inclined to recidivism. Moreover, he usually evinces an unhealthy interest in martial arts, which makes his arrest after his crime contingent upon the presence of at least ten of the boys in blue.

It isn't all grim in prison, though. Sometimes it is fun. My next patient entered my room loudly protesting his innocence.

'I'm not guilty,' he said. 'I've never broke into no houses in Highgate.'

'Oh,' I said. 'Where *do* you break into houses?'

'Islington,' he replied.

'And now you know, sir,' said the prison officer next to me, *sotto voce*, 'why they're in here.'

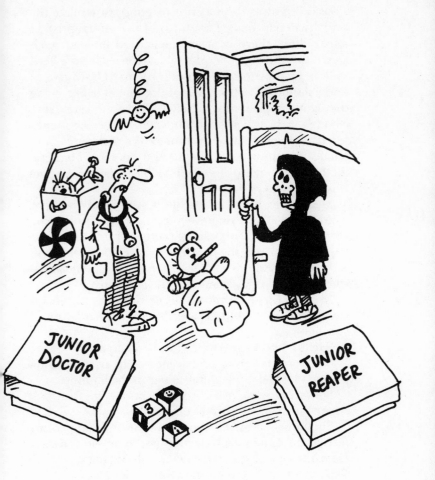

28

I was called away from a crisis meeting last week to the casualty department. I was glad of the interruption, I must admit: there is a certain natural limit to one's interest in the question of new mattresses for the beds in the junior doctors' on-call rooms. Of course, I understand the importance of the matter, sleep being the knitter-up of the ravell'd sleave of care, sore labour's bath, and all that. But when there's no money for mattresses, there's no money for mattresses, and talking about it won't help. And so, like Macbeth, methought I heard a voice cry, 'Sleep no more! The Budget murders sleep.'

Meanwhile, down in casualty a young lady in a red bandanna was spraying everyone in sight with shaving foam. She had bought it, apparently, as protection from the demons which she had recently taken to seeing and hearing everywhere, rather as nervous ladies in violent cities carry tear-gas around in their handbags.

Everyone had retired to a safe distance and it was clearly time for a little leadership, exercised by me. I strode forward.

'Hello,' I said cheerfully. 'I'm Dr Dalrymple.'

She pointed her aerosol at me (ozone friendly, I am glad to say) and applied her finger to the button.

Sticks and stones may break my bones, but foam will never hurt me. I continued my approach.

She punched me hard on the nose and slapped my face. I think she may have reactivated an old fracture, from the time I crashed into a wall during a furious drive to reach a restaurant before it closed.

I had my revenge, however: I ordered her to be held down and injected in the buttock.

I was called to the ward, where another patient awaited me. He was multiply tattooed with symbols of whose meaning and significance he was as perfectly unaware as is the writer of any post-modernist novel of the meaning of the symbols he uses. When I looked at the patient, I could not but think of newsreels of bygone wars: all those patriotic women lining up to donate their rings to the war effort. I pictured my patient – if ever we go to war again – removing the rings from his eyebrows, the upper parts of his ears and his nipples, to help the boys at the front: there were enough of them to pay for an entire campaign, I should have thought.

'What's the problem?' I asked.

'Why do you ask?' he replied. 'What fucker gives a shit?'

'Has it ever occurred to you,' I asked, 'that no one cares because of the way you talk to him?'

'If you'd been through what I've been through . . .' he said.

'Even so,' I said, 'politeness pays.'

'I can't help it.'

I told him that I would continue to see him only on condition that he did not swear or use foul language.

'I'm sorry, doctor,' he said. 'It's just the way I was brought up.'

My plan is to demonstrate to him that, notwithstanding his upbringing, he can control his language; and if he can control that, perhaps he can control other things. Of course, my plan may not work, but if it doesn't – well, to quote my patient, what fucker gives a shit?

29

In my experience, men who kill their wives for the insurance money do so within two weeks of raising the sum assured. This, of course, gives the police a valuable clue as to the identity of the chief suspect in the case, and also as to his motive. It requires, after all, relatively slight knowledge of human nature to put this particular two and two together.

Last week, I was asked to write the annual medical report on a life-sentence prisoner. No one knows why life-sentence prisoners must have such a report prepared on them every year, as if they were old cars undergoing certification of roadworthiness, but it has been decreed by Authority and therefore must be done. I suspect it is one of those make-work regulations which persuade public servants that they are labouring very hard indeed on the public's behalf.

Some years previously, the prisoner, finding himself in an awkward financial predicament, had increased the life insurance on his wife from £90,000 to £270,000. A week later he strangled her, ran from the house, stayed in a nearby hotel for a couple of days, returned home to 'find' her body, and raised a hue and cry. This fits another pattern which has brought itself to my attention: what one might call the *Someone Must Have Killed My Wife Syndrome*. It did not take the police long to work out what had happened. And not surprisingly also, the judge at the trial passed some rather adverse comments on the man's character.

The annual lifer report is supposed to remark not only the prisoner's physical but mental well-being. The latter was presently being attended to by a counsellor, who was helping the prisoner 'come to terms' with his loss: of his wife, I wondered, or his anticipated £270,000? So far, alas, the counsellor had encountered only denial, the omnipresent psychological symptom which requires for its resolution ... further counselling, of course.

The prisoner entered my room with that fixed expression of venom which tells one immediately that he considers himself ill-treated.

We established that his physical health was good, though he didn't much care for prison food. What about his spiritual health? A good barometer of this is usually taken to be the presence of remorse. The received opinion is that the remorseful are less likely to re-offend than the unrepentant, though it can be difficult to distinguish between true remorse and its thespian equivalent. No such problem arose in this case, however.

'Why did you kill your wife?' I asked.

'Me and she wasn't getting on. We was arguing all the time.'

'Any other reason?' I asked mildly.

He thought for a little while, as though searching in the deep recesses of his mind for some recherché fact, like the date of the Treaty of Nerchinsk.

'No,' he concluded.

'The life insurance of £270,000 you took out on her the week before you killed her had nothing to do with it?'

'It may have been a contributing factor,' he conceded broad-mindedly.

'I should have thought it played rather a large, and possibly exclusive, part,' I said. 'I read in your file that that's what the judge thought, too.'

'Well,' he said, 'you could say I was killing two birds with one stone.'

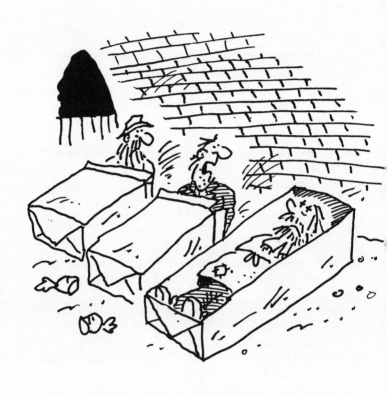

'Old Bert's looking none too well.'

30

I have just returned from the fourth World Conference of Women in Peking, where I was poisoned by piety. It was a great relief to get back to my ward, where people were at least poisoned by para-cetamol or paraquat. In my experience, people who swallow paraquat are generally serious (about death, I mean), though I have known one or two take it for what they supposed were medicinal reasons. Goodness knows what they thought was going on in their insides: they seemed to take the ancient doctrine of the good clear-out to absurd extremes.

Talking of absurd extremes, the conference demon-strated a characteristic of the modern world, namely that its intellectual life consists largely of the solemn enunciation either of the obvious ('girls are the women of tomorrow') or of the obviously wrong ('health is a state of complete physical, mental and social well-being'). How is it that thousands of intelligent people did not notice that this statement, which appeared in the conference document, is drivel? Sometimes I feel like the last person alive who has not been infected by an epidemic virus which affects the brain and turns all thought to mush.

But to return to the really interesting question: why do people poison themselves? Debt, disappointment, depression, drunkenness, fear, jealousy, blackmail, boredom, pique, loneliness, anger, resentment: the whole gamut of unpleasant experience in this vale of tears we call the world.

One of my patients had taken to the pills because the voices told him to do so; another to get the council to place a steel door on her flat, to prevent her jealous, rejected lover from breaking down the wooden door yet again to administer the further beating with which

81

he hoped to win her back to him. In the past, he had broken her arm, he had ruptured her spleen, he had fractured her jaw: am I alone in thinking that a steel door to prevent his ingress should be replaced by a steel door to prevent his egress? How is it possible that a man who has done these things is still walking free?

And then there was a young Indian woman, intelligent and educated, who had agreed to an arranged marriage against her better judgment. Her husband was a mummy's boy, an only son who was the crown prince of the household. In mother's eyes he could do no wrong; and in her eyes also the daughter-in-law, who came to live with them, could do no right. She was treated as a skivvy who was remiss in her duties: she overheard her parents-in-law discussing her, regretting that they had hitched their princely paragon to such a lazy girl.

She was not allowed out of the house under any pretext; she was not allowed to visit her own parents, who in any case would have told her that it was her duty to stay with her husband in order to preserve the family name in the opinion of the community.

My patient took too many pills just to get out of the house for a day or two, the only way she could think of doing so.

As the document produced by the Conference on Women so eloquently puts it:

[Governments should] design and implement ... gender-sensitive health programmes ... that address the needs of women throughout their lives and take into account their multiple roles and responsibilities, the demands on their time, the special needs of rural women and women with disabilities and the diversity of women's needs arising from age, socio-economic and cultural differences, among others, and include women, especially local and indigenous women, in the identification and planning of health-care priorities and programmes ...

82

31

I think I must need counselling. I have arrived at this desperate conclusion because of two posters which appeared recently on the noticeboard of the hospital's Postgraduate Medical Education Centre.

The first of them asks, 'Do you bite your patients' head off?' If the answer is 'Yes, occasionally', the poster recommends that you talk to a friend; but if the answer is 'Yes, all the time', you should consult the Doctors' Counselling Service. (The answer 'No, never' is considered beyond the bounds of possibility, and anyone who replies thus must be a liar.)

The second poster asks, 'Does empathising with your patients depress you?', and makes the same recommendations. I don't know about empathising with my patients, but listening to them certainly depresses me. Surely any man of the most minimal sensitivity would be laid low by what I hear day after day and week in, week out?

But how shall I explain my feelings to my counsellor? And what shall I tell her? Will she understand – empathise with – my view that the misery by which I am surrounded is all the worse for being self-inflicted?

Take the following case. My patient tried to hang himself because he could see no other way out of his predicament. His wife had divorced him on the grounds of unreasonable behaviour – drunken violence etc. – and then remarried him, bearing him three children in quick succession. (The costs of the divorce were borne by Legal Aid, of course.) Then she decided that, because of his continued drinking and violence, she 'needed her own space', with which the council obligingly provided her.

Then she took out an injunction against him – Legal Aid again – but he took no notice of it and assaulted her in her new flat. She called the police, he was arrested, the police filled in their innumerable forms consequent upon an arrest, the case was just about to go to court when she dropped the charges and the happy couple were reunited.

Old habits die hard, however, especially bad ones, and he began to hit her again when drunk – that is to say, seven times a week. She soon told him that she couldn't stand it any more and he had to return to his own flat; but as soon as he got there he decided life was not worth going on with.

'There's nothing left for me, doctor,' he said.

Just as he finished, who should arrive on the ward but his ex-ex-wife. She walked straight up to his bed, flung her arms round him, hugged and kissed him. She had forgiven him everything; she just wanted him back home safe and sound.

Am I unduly harsh in seeing in all this an irresponsible failure on both their parts to take existence seriously? I couldn't help recalling a patient who had been brought to the hospital earlier in the week by a policeman, who had found him in the street with a razor-blade and a cut wrist.

I looked at the wound.

'It's nothing serious,' I said.

'Oh, I know that, doctor,' said the patient. 'I wouldn't do nothing stupid.'

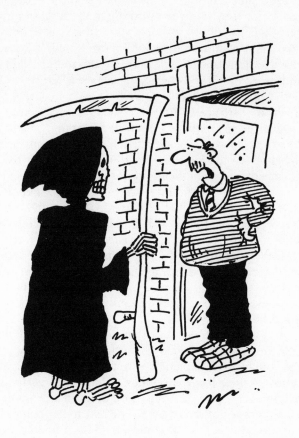

'May I see your ID card?'

32

'If I can't have her, nobody else is going to.'

More sinister words do not exist in the English language, for they serve as a prelude if not always to murder, then usually to a murderous attack. It is not the man's love which is destroyed by the woman's decision to leave him, but his self-love, an altogether different and more dangerous beast, as vicious when wounded as the African buffalo.

To my surprise, however, jealousy was not the motive for my patient's attempt to strangle his wife. This was no common-or-garden asphyxiation, of the tiresome it-was-doing-my-head-in variety; as a consequence of which the man did not even ask that I *sort his head out* so that he should not repeat his strangulations.

It was true that his girlfriend, the mother of his three children, had decided to leave him. They had been together for seventeen years, since they were 15, and she was bored with him. I suspect she was curious as to other men's anatomy. Certainly his conversation was not such as to keep anyone deeply enthralled for decades, even if one counted minutes as years. But he loved her still.

And the problem was that her parents still liked him; he was a steady lad, a good worker and not at all the type to get into trouble with the law. (It was an indication of their low expectations of life, and perhaps of the times we live in, that they defined the good by mere absence of the bad.) So she had to explain to her parents why she was leaving him, when the likelihood was that anyone else she found would be much worse.

She invented a story of his violence towards her: he had beaten her throughout their liaison, she alleged, but now he had tried to strangle her, and that was the final straw.

Naturally, he was displeased by these allegations, coming on top of her decision to leave him. They were completely untrue, and one night the very thought of them drove him to drink. Thereafter, he rose up and attempted to strangle her – a case, I suppose, of life imitating art.

Another patient that day had tried to hang himself because he had done two burglaries, but the police were trying to pin four on him. I told him that I thought the boys in blue would remain unmoved by his protestations of semi-innocence (or semi-guilt, depending on whether by temperament you see the glass half-empty or half-full).

'But that's not all, doctor,' he said.

'What else is there?' I asked.

'I was out of my head at the time.'

'What with?'

'Temarzipan,' he said, meaning temazepam. 'I never go robbing except when I've had temarzipan.'

'Where do you get it from?' I asked.

'A friend.'

Fearing an infinite regress, I pressed my questions no further. Suffice it to say that I have heard tell of wicked old pensioners who sell their prescriptions to young addicts.

'But can't nothing be done to sort my head out?' he asked me when I said I thought the court might view his drug-taking as an aggravating rather than an extenuating circumstance.

For some reason, a single remark from a fellow passenger which a friend and I overheard recently at Moscow airport ran through my head for the rest of the day like a snatch of an unwanted tune: *He should be given a firing squad, as a minimum.*

33

It was a spoonful of tea in which he had let soak a morsel of madeleine which stimulated the efflorescence of Proust's memory. What, in later life, will have the same effect on me?

It will be a smell, an utterly characteristic smell which, once experienced, is never forgotten, and which would open the floodgates of memory in any retired doctor. I refer, of course, to the smell of casualty on a Saturday night, where the air is a stale exhalation of beer, blood and vomit.

Last weekend may have been one of the last occasions when I inspired this gaseous nectar, for two reasons: first I have decided to retire, and second there is a possibility that our hospital will be closed in the near future as an economy measure. After all, if you don't do anything, you can't be accused of inefficiency. Likewise, if there are no out-patient facilities, you can't keep anyone waiting.

The smell was everywhere in the casualty department last Saturday, but was particularly strong in the vicinity of my patient, a youth who had got drunk, vomited and then decided to end it all by cutting his wrists on a number 7 bus, no doubt to the disgust of the other passengers. When I reached him, he was asleep on his trolley. I nudged him awake and wished him good evening, whereupon he belched like the volcanic lake in Cameroon, whose sudden eructation of poisonous gases was responsible for hundreds of deaths.

As for the long-standing rumours that our hospital might close, I first realised they were not entirely without foundation when the whole of the out-patient block was expensively redecorated. This is what boxers and military strategists alike (I believe) call a feint.

Everyone says something like, 'Now they've spent so much money on us, they can't possibly close us down.'

The fools! What do they know of the principles of management? Is it not clear that the way to close down an establishment with the minimum of preliminary fuss is to make everyone who works in it believe that the establishment is sempiternal, and what better way to make them believe that than to refurbish it from top to bottom? A proceeding which appears at first sight to be diabolically incompetent is in fact diabolically cunning.

Of course, in some places the old one-two routine (refurbishment, then closure) doesn't work any more: people eventually grow wise to it. So it has become necessary in the National Health Service to devise a rather more elaborate manoeuvre. A friend of mine, a consultant, reports how even he was taken in lately by the construction of an entirely new hospital wing. Admittedly, it looked a little like a Pizza Hut restaurant, as do all recently erected British buildings, but there was no mistaking the fact that a lot of money had been spent on it.

It came as a shock to him, then, when it was announced that, as an economy measure, the new wing was to be closed down a mere three months after it had opened. Once the shock had abated, however, he was lost in natural admiration. What perspicacity! What foresight! What daring! It is only when one hears such a story that one realises that management is not the mere exercise of common sense, but an art and a science, like medicine itself.

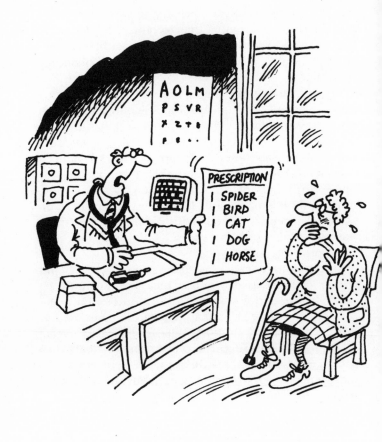

'Take one of these every three hours, old lady.'

34

I don't think I'm an especially delicate plant, but the fact is that it upsets me if more than one patient a day tells me to f— off. One such patient is as much as my attachment to the human race can stand: thereafter, uncharitable thoughts about my fellow creatures begin to supervene, which sour my mood.

Contrary to what many might suppose, I do nothing to provoke these outbursts on the part of my patients. Quite often they address me thus before I have even opened my mouth. And it is unlikely that my body language (to use the modern cant expression for deportment) is so aggressive or offensive that it would explain, much less justify, this manner of speech.

The first such patient last week had taken too much of the drug ecstasy, which in his case seemed to be something of a misnomer, since it made him profoundly miserable and obstreperous. He turned his face to the wall and replied to all questions whatever, from whichever direction they came, with the same obscene expletive, thus displaying what psychiatrists are inclined to call *poverty of speech*, defined in one textbook as speech which 'conveys little information, and tend[s] to be vague, over-abstract . . . repetitive and stereotyped.'

The second patient refused treatment for a potentially life-threatening condition, and I tried to persuade her to accept it. My humanitarian efforts were received with the same implacable hostility, in this case reinforced by the presence of her menacing and unwashed boyfriend, who threatened anyone who approached his beloved with a lawsuit. I knew he was a nasty character, not to be trifled with, because he had drunken-fighter's nose (i.e. broken several times) and two missing upper incisors, a similarly tell-tale sign of habitual inebriated aggression. And he had scars all over his face like ski-tracks in snow.

'I'll have you in court,' he said, waving his index finger in my face.

In the circumstances, it was a relief that my next patient was merely an habitual hypochondriac, who produces symptoms like a conjuror produces rabbits out of a hat. It goes without saying that his real complaint is against life, in all its tedious complexity.

'I've had trouble with Martha, doctor,' he said.

It is a curious fact that many patients think that because *they* know who they are talking about, the doctor must be likewise apprised.

'Who's Martha?' I asked.

'Basically,' replied my patient, 'she's my mother-in-law.'

Her husband, his father-in-law, had just died and there was a family dispute over the tombstone, the choice being between a limestone cross costing £100 or a polished granite affair costing £1,000. My patient favoured the cross, because no one in his right mind would ever visit the grave.

'The cemetery's bad for mugging, you know.'

Naturally, he was distressed by the situation, and it had made all his symptoms worse. He couldn't sleep, either.

'My eyes close, but my inside's open. My wife thinks I'm asleep, but I'm not.'

He had even contemplated ending it all. He would tie a rock to his ankle and jump into the canal.

'And do you know why people end up in the canal, doctor?' he said.

'No, why?' I asked.

'Because doctors aren't understanding enough.'

35

What does experience teach? Only this: that Man (in which designation I include Woman) learns very little from the whole sorry business. Even those who, like me, devote the best part of their lives to the study of human folly in its infinite guises are not necessarily immune from that very foolishness which so distinguishes Man from the animals.

Occasionally, however, one meets somebody who seems to have learnt the beginnings of wisdom from the universal folly by which he is surrounded. For example, only last week I met a man who had come to the conclusion that the currently fashionable way of bringing up children in the quarter of the city from which my hospital draws its patients – and the method by which he himself was brought up – is conducive neither to solid achievement nor even to the most ephemeral happiness. A mother young enough to be your sister, and a succession of temporary stepfathers, is not the best of starts in life.

Unhappily, the mother of his four children was a shrew who combined censoriousness with the grossest irresponsibility and a permanent sense of grievance with violence towards her own children, whom she eventually deserted with a suddenness and finality which was quite startling.

'It's a pity, doctor,' said my patient – though he freely admitted that his wife was a harridan. 'I think a child needs his mother and his father.'

You could have knocked me over with a child protection order.

'For God's sake,' I said, 'don't let a social worker overhear you saying that. Of course, I agree with you, but a social worker would take your children away from you because of your ideas. They'd say your children were in grave danger of growing up judgmental.'

My following patient had led a more conventional life, inasmuch as she was a single mother aged 25 living on the fourteenth floor of a tower block, who had been deserted by the worthless father of her child, whom she still loved though she knew him to be an out-and-out rotter.

Her life was sad and lonely, without interest even to herself. I asked her whether she had been any good at school.

'No, I never went.'

'Why not?'

'I didn't see the point, like.'

I gave her my usual test. I asked her to add eight and seven.

'I can't,' she said, 'because of the drip in my arm.'

'What difference does that make?' I asked.

'I can't use my fingers to count.'

A reading test established that she could pronounce most words of fewer than three syllables, but she could not grasp the meaning of the passage she had just read – in other words, that her educational accomplishments were about average for her age and environment.

'Do you know the dates of the Second World War?' I asked.

'No,' she replied. 'That's one thing I don't agree with, war.'

It seems that, in modern educational theory, to know a fact is to approve of it.

'And what happened in 1066?'

I might as well have asked her the date of the Treaty of Nerchinsk.

'Do you want your son to be educated?'

'Oh yes, doctor. I don't want him to be like me. In fact, I'm going to go to night school myself to learn

English and arithmetic.'

With luck, and much labour (but by no means certainly), she will learn what I knew and took for granted by the age of seven or eight.

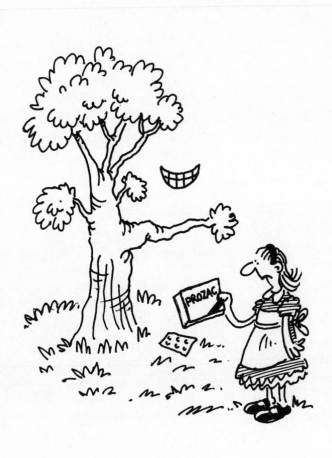

36

There is only one condition less suitable for mankind than slavery and that, of course, is freedom. The main difference between the two conditions is that under slavery it is others who destroy you; while under freedom it is you who destroy yourself. Which is preferable is debatable; but, on the whole, oppression by others annihilates to a slightly lesser degree that illusory hope for the future without which life is almost intolerable.

I am stimulated to these profound but somewhat melancholy reflections by the fate of two young women, the daughters of Indian immigrants, one of whom obeyed her parents and one of whom did not. Both ended miserably, of course: stories round here with happy endings are purely fictional. They belong to Mills and Boon rather than to the narration of Truth.

The obedient girl married her first cousin against her inclinations, the alliance thus cemented raising the status of the family in the eyes of that implacable and unthinking tyrant, the community. But her cousin, the first-born son of his parents who had therefore been raised as a crown prince whose slightest whims were to be attended to at once, turned out to be a vicious scoundrel, who not only beat his newly wedded wife, but his own mother also. The police were sometimes called when things got out of hand, but family honour demanded that no charges were ever pressed.

One might have supposed that, once apprised of the situation, the girl's parents would take her back but, on the contrary, they warned her that if she left the marital home they would ostracise her for having brought shame upon the family. The community which had praised her for her filial obedience would then (rightly, in her parents' view) castigate and scorn her as a prostitute.

The second girl had managed to escape this stulti-fying and cruel atmosphere. She longed for the free-dom English girls had: the very idea of an arranged marriage revolted her. She wanted to find a black-guard of her own, rather than rely upon her parents to do it for her. And who could blame her? It was an act of courage on her part to follow her inclinations and to leave home.

In no time at all, she met her star-crossed tormentor in the kind of nightclub where they don't let you in if you're too well-dressed. A whirlwind romance led within the month to marriage: a marriage which ended in the usual denouement, namely several locks on the front door to keep the ex-husband out and a knife under the pillow in case he should climb through the bedroom window when his urge to beat her up was too strong to be resisted.

Is there then no middle course, I hear you ask, between blind obedience to social custom which cares nothing for the happiness of the individual, and a lone, rudderless voyage on a sea of psychopathy? Only if people were sensible, I reply; and the incontestable fact that history continues to be, indeed, little more than the register of the crimes, follies and misfortunes of mankind would suggest that any hopes in that direc-tion are entirely in vain.

37

An Englishman's home is his castle, wherein no one may enter without permission except the Inland Revenue, the Customs and Excise, burglars, vengeful ex-lovers and neighbours wielding baseball bats. But, in council housing at least, these disturbers of the peace are as nothing compared to the invisible invader brought on wings of vibration for up to twenty-four hours per day. I refer, of course, to music in its louder and more popular forms.

Many people are reduced to fits of murderous or suicidal despair by this curse of the modern age, people who are by no means morbidly hypersensitive to noise, and who themselves are not exactly dormice. Those who complain about it to their neighbours risk death, and are lucky if all they get is a good dose of what is known locally as *verbal*. Neighbours round here are inclined to be what prison officers call *mouthy*.

Of course, people sometimes hear what isn't there. For example, I received a call from the casualty sister last week who informed me that a man had walked through the doors, escorted by two policemen, who had gone to the city centre that morning and found it full of sinners.

'But it *is* full of sinners,' I said.

'I know,' replied Sister. 'But he says he can hear the Holy Spirit as well.'

'What does it say to him?'

'It tells him to spit at policemen.'

This seemed to be carrying the principle of rendering unto Caesar those things which are Caesar's a little far.

But one day this week I was consulted by two patients whose sensations were veridical, and who wished to depart this life because of the music played

99

incessantly by their neighbours.

The first of my two patients wisely took the precaution of sending his wife (who is pregnant) and his first child to his mother-in-law's house before complaining to his neighbour about the volume of music at unearthly hours of the morning. He tried appealing to his neighbour's better nature by telling him that his child needed to sleep and that his wife was pregnant.

'I don't give a f—,' said his neighbour. 'I've got a right to play music if I want to.' And since moderation in defence of human rights is no virtue, he added that he would kill my patient's son if he – my patient – were to complain to the police or to the council.

My second patient had a similar experience when she complained to her neighbour, except that he grabbed her round the throat and banged her head against the wall.

Both patients wanted to move away, of course, but the council considered that they were already adequately housed where they were, inasmuch as they had four walls around them and a roof over their heads which didn't leak in a thunderstorm. Their despair was nearly complete, and they both asked me to write letters to the council on their behalf. They apparently still believed that the council disposed of accommodation where neighbours did not play music at a trillion decibels from midnight to midday.

As I wrote the letters, I thought of the perfect bureaucratic solution to the problem: the Housing Department should make them swap flats.

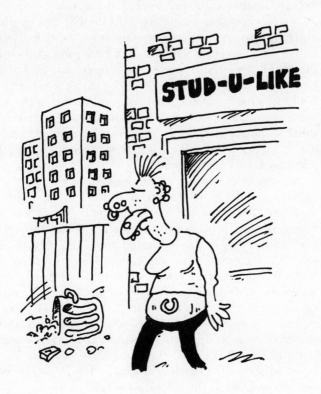

38

These days, like nearly all my patients, I'm tired and lack energy. In fact, I go to bed tired and wake up exhausted. Occasionally, of course, I have some slight excuse for my inertia: last week, for example, I was on duty overnight and found myself called at two in the morning to scour a piece of wasteland about half an hour's drive away, to which a man had gone to spend the night, apparently under the impression that the end of the world was nigh. Why he thought this particularly unattractive corner of the world, with its greasy pond, abandoned perambulators and surfeit of thistles, should be spared the great immolation, I cannot imagine. If the end is nigh, why not just go to bed and wait for it quietly there?

However, one cannot expect logic from a lunatic.

Next morning, or rather a little later the same morning, I was awoken by the hospital. There was a heavy drinker in the ward – a patient, I hasten to add – who was trying to throw himself out of the window to escape an axeman who was coming after him. As it happens, we get quite a few axemen in our ward, but on this occasion it was a purely imaginary one who was causing all the trouble. The windows had been smashed by a similar patient only the week before, and the maintenance department would react rather like Lady Bracknell if they – the windows – were put out again so soon afterwards. Personally, I'm in favour of reinforced glass as the solution to DTs.

On the way into the hospital, I could not help but recall a patient who consulted me earlier in the week. He couldn't sleep, he said, because his mind was 'going ten to the dozen'. That was exactly how my mind was working.

It's odd how patients get the wrong end of the stick

about almost everything. They don't just mix metaphors, they positively mangle them. As for the medical information they're given, they've forgotten it by the time they reach the consulting-room door, and then make something up to tell anyone who'll listen. I've overheard people on trains relaying to each other what the doctor allegedly told them, and it renders newspaper reporting positively accurate by comparison.

And patients, it seems to me, have a very odd set of values. Here again everything is topsy-turvy. One example will suffice. A young man was admitted to our hospital last week having been stabbed in the stomach by his best friend. They had gone to a pub, got drunk and fallen out over a girl. One of them had impugned the other's masculinity, they fought, and a knife was drawn.

Two days later, I was surprised to see the assailant chatting amicably to his victim by his bedside.

'You've forgiven him, then?' I said to the victim.

'Yes,' he replied. 'Mind you, I know we shouldn't have had a fight – but I don't think I deserved to get stabbed.'

'And you,' I asked the assailant, 'what do you think about having stabbed your friend in the stomach like that?'

'I'm gutted,' he replied.

39

The staff of Air France chose the precise moment of my arrival at Charles de Gaulle airport last week to go on strike. I make no claim for a causal connection – but still the coincidence was impressive, and might have powerfully affected someone of less scientific temperament than mine. Instead of brooding upon it, however, I took the opportunity afforded by my longer than foreseen wait for a return flight to these benighted shores to read *Le Monde*.

It was with a certain balefully patriotic satisfaction that I read in that serious, not to say solemn, publication that the back-to-front-baseball-cap and mugging 'culture' (as the promiscuously charitable anthropologists would no doubt call it) now dominates the slums of France. The difference between France and Britain, of course, is that while only a third of France is a slum, two thirds (at least) of Britain is.

Back in the hospital after a short break, I discovered that nothing had changed in my absence, at least not for the better. My first patient, aged 25, had false teeth: not dental decay (fluoride in the water supply having abolished all that), but the violence of her lover. And he had just broken her jaw because the eggs she had cooked for him were not to his complete satisfaction. But she was afraid to leave him because he had threatened to break her mother's legs if she did so.

'Prison's nothing to him,' she said. 'Besides – I know it sounds silly to you, doctor – I love him.'

As for his more serious offences against her, they were so unspeakably awful that I cannot record them here.

My next patient had been prevented by his step-father from attending school between the ages of 6 and 15. He had been continually beaten by him, ostensibly

104

for such reasons as failing to tie his shoelaces in the prescribed fashion, but really to satisfy this latterday Murdstone's desire to beat a fellow human being with utter impunity.

And then there was a girl aged 18, imprisoned, beaten, tortured and repeatedly raped by her 19-year-old boyfriend. I knew her story to be true because I had previously attended the boyfriend's mother and sister, whom he had also beaten savagely. The police have been called to his home more than once, but no charges have been laid: his victims have refused to testify in court against him because flesh is thicker than law, which in any case provides no more protection against violence of this kind than holy water against bullets.

I left the ward with a deep loathing of humanity. Or perhaps it was disgust at my own impotence (and everyone else's, apparently) in the face of this evil. At any rate, that afternoon I was in no mood for prisoners' complaints.

'Doctor,' said the first of them, 'you'll have to give me something to control my temper.'

'Why?' I asked.

'I keep losing it. Last week I poured a saucepan of curry over one of the screws.'

'Was it hot?'

'You mean spicy?'

'No, I meant temperature.'

'No, not very. You know what prison food's like – or perhaps you don't.'

'As a matter of fact I do.'

'Oh do you?' he said, raising an eyebrow. 'Well, anyway, it was only a vegan curry.'

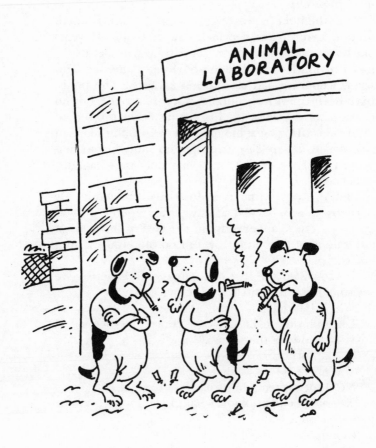

40

There is a group of symptoms, deemed serious by psychiatrists, known as passivity phenomena. The patient no longer experiences his thoughts, volitions or actions as his own, but believes them to be under the direct influence of outside forces, such as other minds, radio waves and cosmic rays. In the words of one textbook, these phenomena represent 'a disturbance in the sense of the integrity of the self'.

This disturbance, it seems to me, is more widespread than the psychiatrists have hitherto acknowledged, and is becoming ever more prevalent. For example, last week I was consulted by two people who were not fully in control of themselves. One lady had resorted to that common expedient, the overdose, calling an ambulance immediately afterwards.

'My doctor made me take it,' she said.

'Oh, really?' I said, most surprised. 'How?'

'He wouldn't give me no sleeping tablets, and I need sleeping tablets to sleep.'

'And then you took the overdose?'

'Yes, he forced me to. I couldn't do nothing else.'

'Let me see if I have understood you correctly. Your doctor refused to give you sleeping tablets, then he grabbed you by the nose, thus causing you to open your mouth in order to breathe, then he stuffed tablets down your throat, and closed your mouth again to make you swallow them?'

She laughed. 'Well, no, not exactly.'

'Then in what sense did he force you?'

'He didn't give me no sleeping tablets.'

Personally I am in favour of giving everybody what he wants, providing only that he takes the responsibility for the consequences. In Third World countries, for example, you can buy powerful cytotoxics over the counter whenever you feel you have a touch of cancer, an excellent system which cuts out the expensive rigmarole of diagnosis.

My second patient with a disturbance of ego boundaries looked a complete mental and physical wreck. He was weak, sallow and thin: every movement appeared to sap his last strength.

'It's the drugs, doctor.'

'Which drugs?' I asked.

'I take everything I can get my hands on.'

Certainly the list he gave me was impressive: black, crack, speed, acid, ecstasy, ice, weed, magic mushrooms and sleepers. And methadone on prescription.

'You know, all this isn't very good for you,' I said.

'I know, doctor, but I've been doing it a long time.'

It is strange how human beings believe that foolishness is extenuated by prolongation.

'It's a pity you ever started,' I said.

'But what else could I do, doctor? I was sent to prison, and prison's awash with drugs, they was all around me.'

'But you didn't have to take them.' This struck my patient as a highly original thought.

I do not mean to imply, though, that people never genuinely lose control of themselves, far from it. It so happens that I was on duty in the evening, and a custody sergeant from a local police station rang to say that they had a drunkard in the cells, but that they feared something was wrong with him. Could I come and examine him?

On the cell walls were scratched desperate messages of love: *Frizz luvs Tracy*, and so forth. There was a terrible smell.

'He defecated in here, doctor,' said the custody sergeant. And then he told me what he did with the products of elimination.

'Not very nice,' I said, wrinkling my nose.

'Average,' said the sergeant, lugubriously.

All the way home a question arose in my mind: what, then, is below average?

41

I went on a long journey by telephone last week. It started with a message in my office on that fiendish modern invention, second in its monstrousness only to the television, the answerphone. Someone who spoke with a nasal whine and who called herself 'the Director of Nursing Quality Assurance' in a neighbouring hospital blathered on about a problem which had arisen there, probably as a result of the habitual negligence of the staff, and asked whether I should be willing to sit as an impartial investigator on the informal commission of inquiry which the hospital was setting up to head off more serious investigations.

Being an obliging sort of chap, especially when it comes to finding fault in others, I thought I should agree. Unhappily, the Director of Nursing Quality Assurance omitted to leave her telephone number, so I had to contact her through her hospital's switchboard.

Having discovered the number of her hospital, I phoned it. After an unconscionable number of rings, a recorded voice welcomed me to St B—'s Hospital, and asked me to hang on while my call was put through to the operator, or alternatively, if I knew the number of the extension I required, I could enter it now. Not being in possession of that invaluable information, I hung on: for a long time, as it happened.

Eventually an operator spoke.

'Hello, St B—'s Hospital.'

'Hello,' I said. 'Could I speak to Miss L—, please?'

'Miss who?'

'Miss L—,' I repeated.

There was a pause of the kind frequently described as pregnant, but in this case there was a miscarriage.

'I've never heard of her. There's no Miss L— here.'

'Yes there is,' I said. 'She's Director of Nursing

Quality Assurance.'

I heard a slight humph, with which I was fully in sympathy, and then a sound like a shuffling of papers. The operator also consulted in a murmur with her colleagues. Then the phone appeared to go dead. After five minutes I replaced the receiver, and started the process again. But I protested when I got through to the operator.

'You cut us off,' she said tetchily.

'I didn't know whether you were still there,' I said. 'I mean, there was no Vivaldi or "Greensleeves".'

'Well, we were still trying for you,' she said. 'Putting you through now,' she added ill-humouredly.

An extension number rang about ten times, and then transferred automatically to another.

'Hello, Mr G—'s secretary.'

'I was looking for Miss L—,' I said.

'Her secretary's on annual leave, I'm afraid, I'm standing in for her,' said Mr G—'s secretary (Mr G— was Director of Nursing Professional Development, incidentally).

'I'd like to speak to Miss L—,' I said.

'She's not here, I'm afraid,' said Mr G—'s secretary.

'Where is she?'

'At the M— Hospital.'

I phoned the M— Hospital.

'Hello, the M— Hospital. How may I help you?'

'I'd like to speak to Miss L—, please.'

'Miss who?'

'Miss L—. She's Director of Nursing Quality Assurance at St B—'s Hospital.'

'Never heard of her.'

There was more rustling of paper, and more murmurous conversation with colleagues.

'She's in a meeting.'

'Could you get her out of the meeting?' I asked.

'We don't know where it is.'

'Then how do you know she's in it?' I asked. The deep epistemological import of my question, with its undertones of Bishop Berkeley, was entirely lost.

'We can't find her.'

But I found her next day, and expressed the view most forcefully that it would have been better if she had cut the cackle on my answerphone and just told me her telephone number and when I could reach her there.

'But are you still willing to help, doctor?' she asked.

'Of course,' I said.

The following day, she called me.

'After your outburst of temper yesterday,' she said, 'we don't want you any more.'

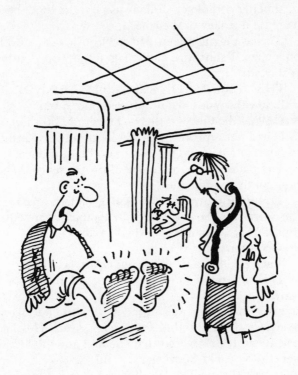

'They're injuries sustained from trying to get to Casualty.'

42

No sooner had I arrived in the hospital one day last week than I was asked to go to the casualty department. A young man had been brought in not long before who had taken too many sleeping pills. The hospital being completely full, as usual these days, he was lying on a trolley in the corridor.

He was deeply asleep. He smelt unwashed and had on a black T-shirt with a long legend in white lettering. It started:

THE TEN GREATEST FUCKS IN THE WORLD

Below this was a list numbered one to ten.

1. What the fuck was that? – Mayor of Hiroshima.

I shall not reproduce the list in its entirety. Suffice it to say that No. 1 was the most tasteful of the ten.

The patient being unaware of my presence, I shook him gently to wake him.

'Fuuuuuuuuuuuuuuuuck,' he groaned, expanding the word as a South American football commentator on the radio expands the word 'goal'.

'Good morning,' I said.

'Fuck off,' he said, a little wider awake.

This, of course, put me in a good mood for the wards.

First on the left was a girl of 12 who had taken an overdose of her mother's antidepressants. Her father had recently discovered that she had gone to bed with her 19-year-old boyfriend, and had accordingly informed the police. The boyfriend and some of his mates (as she called them) had come to the house and had broken his legs with baseball bats to encourage him to withdraw the charges.

Next to the young overdoser was a slightly older overdoser. Her ex-husband was giving her trouble again: he had put an axe through her front door the day before. He was not a pleasant man: he had, among other things, locked her in a cupboard for days on end.

'Once he held me by the ankles out of the eleventh-floor window of our flat, shouting, "What's it like to die, bitch?" '

'You didn't leave him afterwards?'

'No.'

'Why not?'

'I loved him. Besides, I didn't know no different.'

At first I was incredulous. How could anyone know no different? Then I looked at her address: a tower block to which I had once been called because a resident had abseiled down the front of the building from his flat on the fifteenth floor. It was feared that there was something medically wrong with him.

I went up to his flat. He opened the door. All was darkness inside. The rooms were bare and cold, but in the centre of the largest of them was a crude iron brazier, with some dying red embers. The abseiler took cocaine and used all his income to buy it. Now he was burning his furniture to keep warm.

'Why did you abseil down the building?' I asked.

'I wanted to test my escape route,' he replied, 'in case of fire.'

No wonder someone in the block considers it perfectly normal to be suspended by the ankles from the eleventh-floor window.

My next patient in the ward had also been locked in a cupboard by her husband – who was a policeman. He wanted to make sure she did not misbehave while he was out on the beat.

'Why haven't you left him?' I asked her.

'I have, doctor,' she replied. 'Lots of times.'

43

I suppose every scribbler, no matter how much of a hack he may be, secretly harbours a desire for a measure of literary immortality. To be remembered for a book – no, for a sentence or even a single phrase – is a better fate than the complete oblivion in the minds of the still living to which most of us are consigned soon after our deaths.

Well, my recent researches have proved conclusively that literary immortality is not all it's made out to be. If it's fame you want, you're better off with football.

Take Shakespeare, for example. I dare say everyone will agree that he is as immortal as it is possible to be, this side of a cryonics laboratory in California. Yet even in the land of his birth his name does not ring a bell in every mind. Quite the contrary.

Last week I was consulted by two pleasant young men, who were clean, polite and law-abiding. They had never truanted from school and, though they were clearly not of giant intellect, they were not of defective intelligence either. I suspected, however, that their formal education had not been rigorous and my suspicions were soon confirmed by a little test.

Neither was able to add 9 to 12, though one was pleased when I told him that his answer, 20, was nearly correct. Their knowledge of geography was limited: neither knew the capital of Russia, and one thought the capital of Germany was Denmark. Their knowledge of history was not extensive: neither knew when the Second World War started and one thought it finished in the 1950s. Neither knew when the First World War took place, not even to within the nearest 100 years. Neither knew what had happened in 1066. When I asked one of them what he knew of Stalin, he replied, 'I haven't heard of that.'

He had heard of Hitler, however.

'He was a German person who killed all the Jews.'

As to prime ministers, they could name only Mr Major and Mrs Thatcher: they said they were too young to remember any others.

I asked about Shakespeare. Both their brows furrowed, and both denied acquaintance with him. I asked them to think again, to search in the innermost recesses of their minds.

After an intense struggle, one of them muttered, 'He prances about in an outfit, doesn't he?' Having been educated by teachers who believed in the sanctity of self-expression, he was unable to explain himself further. This was the unsmashable atom of his knowledge of Shakespeare.

The other asked for a clue.

'He was a writer,' I said.

'Was he?' said the young man, genuinely surprised. 'I thought he was a composer.' Finally, something stirred in his mind, as slowly as a tectonic plate. 'Oh yeah, he done all them plays.'

Now what I should like to know is this: how have institutions of learning been created which impart so little knowledge to children in eleven years of tuition? Who is responsible for leaving children with no more bearings in the world than if they had been lowered alone in a canoe into the vastness of the Pacific? And why have the British people not risen up to slaughter those responsible in their beds, as they so manifestly deserve?

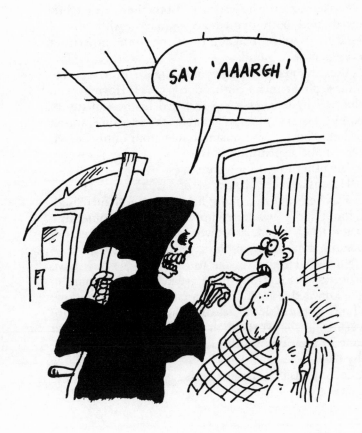

44

I returned home recently after a short break away from my patients – any break from my patients is short, of course, however long it may be. I suppose I should not have been surprised or disappointed to discover that in my absence nothing much had changed in the hospital or in the country as a whole, though the underside of the desk in my office had in the meantime acquired some used chewing gum. I should like to inform the ruminant interloper that he may reclaim his property on any weekday between 9 a.m. and 1 p.m.

My first patient was a 17-year-old girl, wearing too much lipstick, who had taken the drug Ecstasy in the sleazy hotel in which Social Services had placed her after she decided that she had had enough of her parent. I asked her what she wanted to do in life.

'Nothing,' she said.

Welcome to Britain, I thought.

'Do you mean there's nothing you want to do, or you want to do nothing?' I asked. 'There's a slight difference, you know.'

But it was too slight for her comprehension.

'Well, anyway,' I said consolingly, 'I should imagine you'll achieve your ambition.'

My second patient after my return to these islands was an alcoholic who had been mugged in the city one night the week before, and had been stabbed all over, apparently for the fun of it.

His was a lamentable life story. At the age of 9 he was sent to children's homes because his drunken and violent father was considered a threat to his well-being. At the age of 16 he entered on a life of crime, and spent most of the next twenty years in prison. The last ten years had been forensically blameless.

'I didn't mind prison in them days,' he said. 'I weren't afraid of it. I didn't mind being told what to do. In fact I liked it, but I wouldn't like it now.'

Unfortunately, his accretion of wisdom in the intervening years was only marginal. He used his new-found freedom to acquire cirrhosis of the liver.

His brother, a few years younger than he, was an alcoholic also. Four weeks ago, at the age of 38, he died of a cerebral haemorrhage. Since that time, my patient had tried to hang himself and gas himself, he had jumped out of a first-floor window, thus spraining both his ankles, and had taken an overdose twice a week.

On the day his brother died, his daughter, aged 17, gave birth to a baby.

'What did you think of that?' I asked.

'I was really proud of her,' he said.

'And what about the father?' I asked.

'Oh, he fucked off.'

'What did you think of him?'

'If I found him I'd punch him in the face.'

'Why?'

'Well, I always thought the blood on the walls and floor in her flat was because of her periods, but it was because he was beating her up. He used to drink. I didn't know that. My daughter never told me.'

'And your daughter: what does she think?'

'She says she'd like more children. She's really happy with the baby, like.'

45

There is no doubt that Mr Lilley, the Minister for Social Justice, is putting fear into the hearts of the malingering classes. I discovered this while a prominent member of these classes, a patient of mine, aged 56, was explaining to me why it was that he made love to Iris at every opportunity which presented itself, even though she lived in a home, made love to lots of other men, was 60 years old and wouldn't be allowed out again if the nurses discovered what she was doing during her so-called walks.

'I'm not a pervert, I just can't help myself, doctor,' he said. 'Besides, I like it. That's why I knock her off, as they call it. It's natural: you can't stop a bird eating worms.'

But the real reason for his behaviour ran deeper (of course, it always does). The fact was that his wife had never satisfied him sexually, not in thirty-six years of marriage.

'She sits at night with babies' nappies on, you have to take them off before you can do anything. It's not very inviting.'

I was beginning to feel slightly uncomfortable: there are, after all, some confidences of which one would rather not be the repository.

'I want someone to love me like they do on the telly or the films, not like my wife loves me. She just lies on the bed and tells me in the middle of it that there are some cobwebs on the ceiling, or sometimes she mentions Mr Lilley's new system of invalidity benefit – incapacity benefit, I think he calls it – and it puts me off, like, I get all nervous and I can't go on.'

I must confess that, experienced as I am at listening impassively to the utmost absurdity, I laughed. Until then, I had never thought of government ministers as bromides, rather as soporifics.

'My wife doesn't understand me, doctor,' he continued. 'She doesn't understand my need for sex. That's why I'm always after Iris, I'm just like any other man. And I'd tell her to her face if she was here, in front of you, like.'

I said nothing. With only the faintest of discernible movements, I moved my shirt cuff back so that I could glance at my watch. I suspected that my patient's time was up.

'Only if I don't have the sex what I need, doctor, I begin to get a bit up-pent, and then I spring like a big rat. You're not like me, are you, doctor?'

'Er, no,' I said, reluctant as ever to answer a patient's question.

'I don't suppose you've ever done the opposite of what you really wanted to do, like me. You can control yourself, because you're a doctor. You're not like me, you think before you act.'

'Generally, yes,' I said.

Then he thought of a solution to his problems. He wanted me to admit him to hospital for four years, until he could draw his old-age pension.

'After all,' he said, 'there's patients in that hospital who aren't no worse than what I am. They're like children, only they've got adults' minds.'

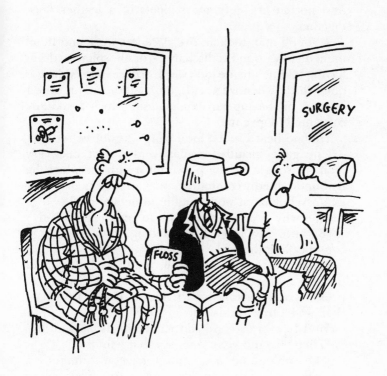

46

Wrongdoers and lawbreakers used to seek sanctuary in the church; nowadays they seek it in the hospital. It isn't only the police they wish to avoid: it is each other. And not surprisingly, for patients of a feather flock together.

A young man took an overdose last week and then, immediately upon his discharge from hospital (without having told us why he took the overdose, indeed he got quite shirty when we asked), took another. This time I insisted on having an explanation, which he kindly consented to give me.

He had heard that a local gang was out to get him. As the gang included a man who was at that very moment sought by the police for a murder which he had undoubtedly committed, my patient's anxiety was, as a psychoanalyst would put it, understandable.

'And why does the gang want to get you?' I asked.

'Because my sister keeps telling them that I go round calling them black cunts.'

What? In the multicultural, multiracial Britain of the late 20th century? When – as the Transylvanian peasants asked about the activities of Count Dracula – shall we be free of this evil?

'And I never even called them bastards black cunts.'

'Then why did your sister say that you did?'

'She can't stand me.' And I have to admit that, superficially at least, he was not an attractive personality. 'She wants me out of the way.'

I admired her brilliant scheme to rid herself of her brother, though I refrained from expressing my admiration to him.

'She's only my half-sister, like.'

'Which half?'

'You what?'

'Do you have the same mother or the same father?'

'I don't know.'

Fortunately it was lunch-time, which brought my investigations of the mating habits of the British to a close. I had to attend an important meeting with the managers.

'It has come to my notice,' said the Deputy Director of Patient Services (whatever they may be), 'that there have been four fires on the wards in the last three weeks. They were started by patients smoking in bed. Eighty per cent of fire deaths in this country are caused by people who smoke in bed. The situation is even more dangerous now than it used to be since ...' He paused for a moment, to consider whether it was wise to continue. '... since the installation of the fire doors in the corridors.'

It is true that they are rather stiff and might pose a problem to someone with, say, a stroke or pneumonia.

'We must do something about it.'

'Asbestos sheets,' I muttered.

'Sprinkler systems over the beds,' suggested my colleague to my left. 'Activated by cigarette smoke.'

'Unfortunately, our patients are not always co-operative or understanding. Indeed, when asked to stop smoking in bed, they often become abusive or threatening. There have been two assaults on the nurses when they were asked to extinguish their ciga-rettes or go outside to smoke.'

It was then that the solution occurred to me in a flash. Let the punishment fit the crime: an *auto-da-fé* in front of the hospital. As a fund-raising event it could hardly be bettered: the British have always been rather keen on public executions.

'I have appointed a subcommittee,' said the Deputy Director of Patient Services, interrupting my reverie, 'and asked them to produce a Draft Arson Policy by next week.'

47

Every time I enter the prison of late I wonder, the feeling of doom upon me, how I myself should survive a prison sentence. I think on the whole that it would not be insupportable on two conditions, the first that I should be innocent of whatever it was that I was charged with (just deserts being so much more burdensome, psychologically speaking, than unjust ones), and the second that I were placed in solitary confinement.

Not everyone would agree, of course: not for nothing is human variety infinite. A patient of mine, released a month ago from prison after a twelve-month stretch, complained that he still sweated heavily at night.

'I think it's me nerves, doctor.'

Long acquaintance with the human race made me suspect alcohol.

'I don't think so, doctor. I admit I used to drink heavy, but I haven't had nothing to drink since I left prison – not what you'd call a good drink, like. I'd of thought all the beer would of come out of me by now.'

I asked him how prison had been.

'Terrible, doctor. It was my first time.'

'What was terrible?'

'Knowing you hadn't of done it, doctor.'

'You were innocent?'

'Yes, but I took the rap and done the time.'

'Did you know who did it?'

'Yes.'

'Why did you take the rap, then?' I asked.

'Well, I know a lot of lads, like, doctor, and you don't grass on them, not to the police.'

'Honour among thieves?'

'Sort of.'

'And what would have happened if you'd grassed on them?'

126

'I'd of bin in a coffin by now, doctor, or I'd of lost my legs.'

It was reassuring to learn that in some circles of society, at least, the belief in the efficacy and moral justification of deterrence and retribution has not yet quite evaporated.

'There was another banger, doctor,' said my patient.

'Banger?' I enquired.

'A banger, doctor: something what does your head in.'

'And what was it?'

'I was locked up in my cell all day. Nothing to do but look at the walls.'

'Didn't you have anything to read?'

'I can't read and write, doctor.'

I gave him a test. He didn't even know his alphabet.

'I've often thought it would be great to be able to read a newspaper.'

I confess that even my hard heart contracted in sorrow.

'Didn't your teachers ever notice?' I asked.

'I bunked off, doctor. And I always got my class-mates to do my work. I wish I hadn't of done it now.'

'Yes,' I said. 'It was a mistake.'

'It's always stopped me getting a job, not being able to read and write – that's why I turned to the life of a villain.'

'Would you like to learn?' I asked.

'I'd love to, doctor.'

I phoned the local adult education office.

'I'll put you through to the department which deals with people with supported learning.'

Was I hearing aright? I think so.

'Hello, I'm Jenny. I deal with people with supported learning.'

I explained my patient's problem.

'And is he abled?'

'Do you mean, can he walk?'

'Yes.'

'In that case, he is abled.'

When I put the phone down, my patient asked whether I thought he might be sweating at night because one of his neighbours was out to get him.

'You see, doctor,' he said, 'he's got a denvetta against me.'

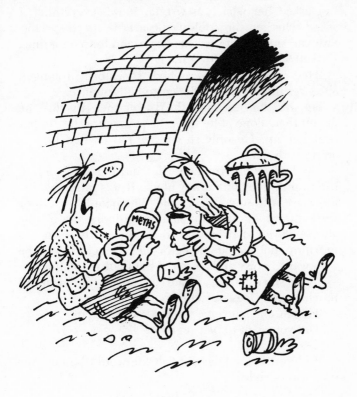

'Shall I be single mother?'

48

I was in Casualty last week when a woman who had tried to hang herself was brought in. I do not think her effort was a very concerted one: her 4-year-old son managed to stop her before she could kick the stool away. The little hero was then packed off to a neighbour's while mama received medical attention.

I asked her what was wrong. It was everything. I asked whether she couldn't be a little more specific. She said she hadn't seen her boyfriend for a long time. I asked what he did for a living.

'He's a burglar,' she replied. His more prolonged absences usually denoted a custodial sentence.

He was the best man she'd ever met. By this she meant that, alone of her male acquaintance, he did not beat her up. He only shook her hard when he was angry with her.

She had other problems. She and her son lived on the twelfth floor of a tower block. It was miserable living there with so young a child. The people next door were always arguing and slamming doors, the people above played their music so loudly at three in the morning that the people below her thought it was she who was so noisy and were constantly threatening her.

'Your son's father,' I said tentatively and without much hope. 'Does he help?'

'He left me before he knew I was pregnant.'

'Did you want to be pregnant?'

'Yes.'

'Did you know how difficult life would be on your own with a child?'

'Yes, I've had three kids before, doctor.'

'What happened to them?'

'They was took away from me because I come from a broken home.'

More recently, she had made enemies at her local pub. She was anxious about it because a woman had been murdered there not long before.

'I was there one night when the windows went in,' she said.

'The windows went in?' I said.

'Yes, all of them.'

'How did they go in? Was there an earthquake?'

'Someone smashed them, like.'

And what had happened then?

'I don't remember – I'd had a bit to drink. They say I started screaming. The barman said, "Oi you, get out of this effing pub." Then they say that I started on him. He reckons that I showed him up in front of his friends. That's why he came after me and beat me up in the street. He said that when this murder's died down, he's coming for me properly.'

'What's he like, this barman?'

'I've heard he likes hitting women, but when it comes to men he needs a friend or a weapon. He won't fight hand to hand.'

I asked her how she thought I could help her.

'Everything I do seems to fail. I want a new life.'

'How will you get it?'

'I want some help with moving.' That is to say, she wanted me to write to the Housing Department to say that she should be moved for medical reasons (she had asked for a transfer three years ago). I told her that all public housing in the city was the same, and that she should not expect a new life to emerge automatically from such a move.

'And I need help with my finances. I've never been no good with my finances.'

In short she needed a different future, a different present and a different past. She needed to have been born someone else: one of the treatments not available on the NHS.

49

I remember as a child hearing my elders and betters say that accidents, such as plane crashes, come in threes. I still don't know whether they were right, but what I can say with some authority is that maltreated women appear on my ward in threes.

The first of last week's crop was a lady whose boyfriend of two years was the insanely jealous type. He cross-questioned her about where she had been and what she had done, even if she had left the house for only five minutes; he regarded all telephone numbers with the utmost suspicion, searched her bag for evidence of her infidelity and so forth. This behaviour is so common as to be almost normal; but where my patient's boyfriend out-Othelloed Othello, as it were, was in his method of securing her fidelity during his absence for the day. He handcuffed her left wrist to her right ankle.

When she told her father, a respectable man, and he protested to the boyfriend, the latter replied in that charming tone of voice which I know so well, 'You don't frighten me. I can pay twenty pounds and have you killed.'

The second maltreated woman was a young Muslim lady whose parents had taken her recently to Pakistan. They had never permitted her to attend school for any length of time, though secretly she wanted to go to university, because they feared it would corrupt her. She attended school only long enough to keep the school inspectors at bay.

When she arrived in Pakistan, it was announced that she was engaged to be married – next day. The groom was a young man brought up in her household whom she had supposed until then to be her brother. In fact, he was her first cousin. When she said she did not want

132

to marry him, her father beat her with a stick and stamped on her chest. Then he almost suffocated her by sitting on her.

She insisted, however, that she would not marry her fiancé. Her father then threatened to divorce her mother, which in the circumstances would have left her destitute and with an abominable public reputation. My patient surrendered to the blackmail.

After the wedding, the happy couple could not make love, as it seemed almost incestuous to them to do so. But the relatives on both sides were aware of this reluctance, and were moreover impatient for an addition to the family, and so they locked them in a room together for ten days. Still nothing happened; the relatives installed a tape-recorder and said that if at the end of a further period they were not satisfied that intercourse had taken place, they would adopt other, sterner measures.

Autres temps, autres moeurs.

And last, though not necessarily least, was an overdoser whose second husband, like her first, was a drunk. She told me how he had one day tried to strangle his stepdaughter, her 15-year-old daughter by her first marriage.

'That was because you said I fancied her sexually,' interposed the husband.

'Then when I tried to stop you, you strangled me. I went unconscious, doctor.'

'But it was only a one-off.'

'That's true, doctor,' she said in his defence. 'And he only drinks for socialism.'

Drinkers of the world, unite! You have nothing to lose but your shakes!

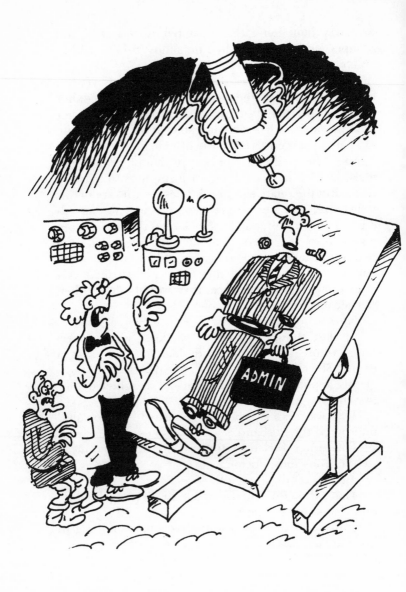

'I, Doctor Frankenstein, will create the ultimate monster.'

50

I was listening to Radio Three on my way to work last week. It is the only radio station I ever listen to, not only because of the music, but because it is entirely Prime Minister-free. Whenever I hear our leader's voice, I begin to empathise with my patients when they say that their heads just went. If I were to hear the PM while driving, I'm sure I should drive straight into a wall or run someone over. Poor chap, he probably means quite well.

I arrived at my hospital to the sound of a Haydn quartet. I was thinking what a piece of work is a man! How noble in reason! How infinite in faculty! In form, in moving, how express and admirable! In apprehension, how like a god! The beauty of the world! The paragon of animals!

Of course, I deal more with the quintessence of dust end of the market.

Awaiting me in my ward was a young lady who wanted to do herself in with some pills. She changed her mind, and called an ambulance immediately on swallowing them. This is so common a pattern of behaviour that I sometimes wonder whether the instructions on the packet do not tell the purchaser to take twenty of the pills and then dial 999.

She had wanted to die because her boyfriend, whom she loved, left her a few months ago.

'Why did he do that?' I asked.

'He thought I was having an affair with his best friend.'

'And were you?'

'No.'

'Was he the jealous type, then?'

'He was a little possessive.'

'Was he violent? Did he ever, for example, hit you?'

'Not very often.'

'Injure you?'

'Broken ribs.'

'Punch?'

'Kick.'

'You were already on the ground?'

'No, I was standing.'

'Ah, he's martial arts trained.'

'Yes.'

'They always are.'

I tried to encourage her to see his desertion more as a lucky escape than as a catastrophe. Even as we spoke (I said) he was probably bashing her successor in his affections.

'No, he knew he had a problem and wanted counselling for it.'

News travels fast on the concrete jungle telegraph, and who should turn up a couple of hours later but the paragon of animals himself. The hair on his head was shaved, except for a ponytail at the back. In his eyes there was a feral look. He reminded me a little of the cats I had seen as a student of physiology, whose heads were shaved and into the amygdala of whose brains were inserted electrodes which, when stimulated, produced a ferocious but undirected and meaningless outburst of rage.

He had several deep scars on his forehead, from smashing his head against the wall when he was angry and there was no one to hit except himself.

'I just lose it,' he said. 'My head goes.'

I suspected his education had not been altogether a success.

'I got all my exams and everythink,' he said.

I gave him my usual little test. I asked him to read a passage, he having claimed to be able to read fluently. He read several lines with the difficult words left out.

'What did it mean?' I asked.

He had no more idea than if it had been written in an ancient holy language whose script he could decipher, but of the meaning of whose words he was completely ignorant – Hebrew, say, or Church Slavonic.

He had passed a public examination in English.

I asked about arithmetic, and he was the second 20-year-old in a week who did not know what arithmetic meant. But he had passed a public examination in maths, he told me.

'Six times nine?' I asked.

He was the tenth such youth, not of subnormal intelligence, this month not to have known.

'I'd have to work it out,' he said.

When I left the ward, he and his girlfriend were reconciled and were cuddling on the bed.

51

Why do people turn to crime? It is difficult to meet so many criminals and not to ponder this vitally important question. Last week, as I was reading in the *British Medical Journal* that smokers have been granted legal aid so that they may sue the tobacco companies for all their ailments, I suddenly was in receipt of a blinding illumination into the cause of crime: smoking.

Only a third of the British population smokes, yet virtually 100 per cent of criminals do so. The next time I entered the prison, I checked that my insight was not the result of mere observational bias by asking a few officers for their estimate of the percentage of cons who smoked. All of them had difficulty recollecting any who didn't. And what is more, they all smoked before they ever came to prison.

Sceptics among my readers might object that, since both smokers and criminals are drawn predominantly from the lower classes, the association between smoking and crime is merely an effect of social class. To which I reply the following:

i) The statistical association between smoking and crime is much stronger and more exact than that between social class and crime, *ergo* social class has nothing to do with it and

ii) In any case, it is much more plausible that indulgence in an expensive habit such as smoking should cause poverty than that poverty should cause an expensive habit such as smoking.

Of course, a scientific pioneer such as myself does not expect to be believed straight away: did they not mock Mesmer and Gall (the founder of phrenology)? But let me assure any householder who has been burgled and is eligible for legal aid that I am prepared to appear on his behalf as an expert witness (legal aid

138

fees £500 per day, plus travel and other reasonable expenses) if he sues the tobacco companies for having promoted burglary through smoking. I also have a friend who is willing to appear, two opinions being better than one.

Contrary to what the layman might expect, flashes of illumination such as mine are very tiring. As soon as it had been vouchsafed me, I felt I wanted to go to sleep. I understood at last what the mother of a patient of mine, a very studious boy, meant when she told him it was bad for him to think so much because he might wear his brain out.

Another of my patients, rather less studious, asked me whether he could have something to make him relax.

'I don't want to think no more, doctor. I could do with a vacation from my mind.'

But to return to the question of legal aid. There is obviously no end to the suits which could justifiably be brought. For example, last week in the prison a newly remanded burglar came into my room clutching his arm, which had been rather badly bitten.

'I'm told I could sue the police for this,' he said, waving his arm in front of me like a trophy.

'Why?' I asked.

'It was a police dog what done it.'

'And what were you doing?'

'Running away.'

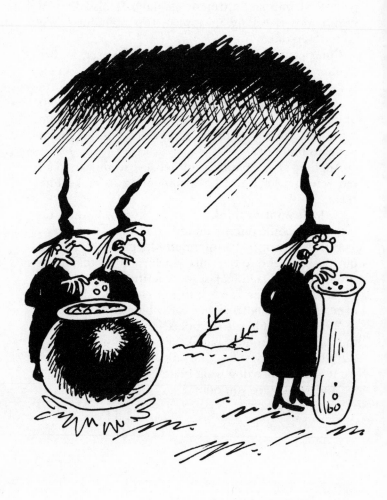

'She's gone into pharmaceuticals.'

52

I visited a different prison last week, situated in one of those small, ancient and delightful English cathedral cities, where all the youths suffer from acne, look stupid and take amphetamines, and where the architectural prospect was modernised and improved during the 1960s and 1970s by the construction and artful placement of a concrete multistorey car park and a tower block or two.

I went by train, for I have reached a time of life when to drive long distances is irksome to me. In theory, at least, one can read on the train, or could if it weren't for the chatter of other passengers. All small talk is small, of course, but that of passengers on British Rail is positively microscopic.

On my arrival at the station at which, according to the conductor, 'this train terminates' (which for some reason put me in mind of Arnold Schwarzenegger), I could not help but notice the general tenor of the first four posters which I passed as I walked along the platform. They seemed to be in ascending order of seriousness. The first of them asked how you would look if you were caught travelling on a train without a ticket. The second drew attention to the existence of the British Transport Police, 'Serving the Railway Community'. The third warned prospective assaulters of British Rail staff that if they acted upon their nefarious inclinations, they might get a heavy fine or imprisonment (or, knowing the courts these days as I do, neither). And finally, there was a minatory exhortation in red lettering:

'BOMBS – BE ALERT.'

Whether it was the bombs or the public who were thus enjoined to caution was not stated.

Evidently, this cathedral city was an evil place.

141

And of course it was a grievous bodily harmer whom I had come to see. His lawyer had wondered (at public expense, naturally) whether his violence could be construed as an epileptic, and therefore medical, phenomenon.

'I'll just produce the body for you, sir,' said a prison officer, which was prison argot for telling the prisoner to enter my room.

I was surprised by the young man's diminutive size: he seemed too small to have harmed anyone. However, like Douglas Bader, he had overcome his disability by sheer will-power. Not that he admitted that he was by nature violent: only a handful of his many offences had involved violence. Besides, he said (somewhat contra-dicting himself), what else could you expect coming from his environment?

He had a point. His father was drunken and aggres-sive, and had been in jug himself. As for his school, he was bullied there because of his small size and because he came from a different council estate from the rest of the pupils – if that is quite the word for them. Every week he was dragged across the playground by the hair, and once the biggest bully in the school announced that he was going to give him a 'posting'.

'What's that?' I asked naively.

'They take you and ram your balls against a post.'

'What did you do?'

'I head-butted him.'

'What happened then?'

'I had to see the headmaster.'

'What did he say?'

'He said it was about time.'

His latest offence was different, however. He had been rat-arsed, he said, at what the lawyers call the material time. He hadn't meant to put his victim into the intensive care unit of the local hospital for several weeks.

'Him and me was mates. It just happened, like.'

53

They say that love is blind, but round here it's a deaf mute as well. Perhaps that's just as well, considering the sensory experience available to most of the local population.

I walked on to the ward last week to find it full of overdosers. One of them was a pretty young woman. I asked her why she'd done it.

'Life in general,' she said, poutingly. 'It's got on top of me.'

Long experience has taught me that Hell is in the detail. And to those who seek the cause of a woman's misery, I offer the following maxim: *cherchez l'homme*.

The man in question had been released from prison two months earlier, after a two-year sentence for having carried on what she called 'his trade', namely demanding money with menaces. I asked whether he had ever been violent towards her.

'A few times, yes,' she said.

'Has he ever injured you seriously?' I asked.

'Once he put my head through a glass door and rubbed my neck on the broken bits. My blood vessels was cut, they thought I wouldn't live. I was in hospital for five weeks afterwards.'

'The police were not involved? They knew nothing about it?'

'No.'

'And you still love him?'

'Well, yes I do. I'm no angel, doctor, I've even attacked him with a knife.

'Is he jealous and possessive, by any chance?'

'Yes, very.'

'So of course he's asking you what you did while he was in prison?'

'Yes, he's asking me all the time, he never believes

143

what I tell him. It's driving me mad.'

'He accuses you?'

'Yes.'

'And doesn't allow you out on your own?'

'Yes. And he doesn't like it if I talk to other men.'

'And he asks you where you've been and what you've done?'

'Yes.'

'And does he say, "If you tell me the truth about the time I was in prison, I won't ask you again, and I'll treat you as if nothing happened"?'

'Yes.'

'Can I give you a word of advice? Confess to nothing, admit nothing. Don't fall for the idea that if you tell him something, it'll clear the atmosphere. He'll kill you instead.'

'I know that, doctor, I'm not that stupid.'

I had no more questions. She asked me whether she needed counselling.

'Yes, if someone with gas gangrene needs hypnotherapy.'

I was about to leave her when she asked me to stay.

'I had an abortion just before he come out of prison, doctor. It wasn't his, of course.'

'Of course.'

'But now I need the six-week examination afterwards, and I can't go to my own doctor.'

'Why not?'

'Because he'd come with me and ask what it was for.'

'So you want it in the hospital?'

'If it's possible, doctor.'

'And that's why you took the overdose? So that you could have an examination while he's not here?'

'That's right, doctor. You see, it hurts when I make love to him.'

As I walked away from her bed, I realised that I had heard a subtle argument in favour of conjugal visits for prisoners. And then a few lines from Emily Dickinson ran through my head:

Tell all the Truth but tell it slant—
Success in Circuit lies—
Too bright for our infirm Delight
The Truth's superb surprise.

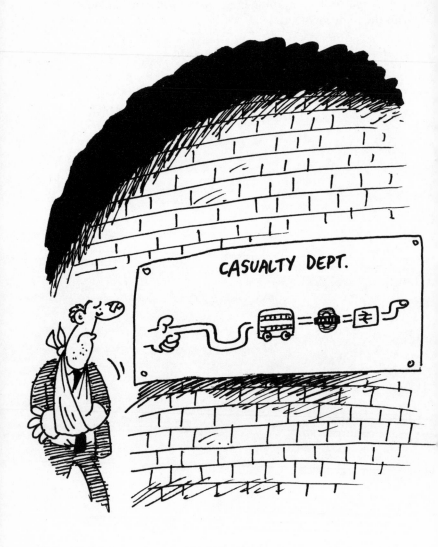

54

It has long been denied by many eminent people, professors among them, that there is any philosophical justification whatever for the practice of punishment. I do not count myself as altogether a sadist, but this view of the ethical impermissibility of punishment, based no doubt on the patently false premise of the natural goodness of man, seems to me absurd. It is fear, after all, which makes the world go round.

The police, alas, have gone over in their entirety to the psychotherapeutic view of life, namely that to understand all is to heal all. The line dividing the police from psychotherapists is now a fine one: they are social workers in uniform.

A patient of mine, a woman in her thirties, was recently mugged by two schoolboys aged 14. In the process she received minor injuries: cuts and bruises. Amazingly, the police caught the two giant brats, and gave them what is now the standard admonishment not to repeat their behaviour.

A week later, my patient found herself the object of unsolicited attentions. First the school from which the two brats truanted sent her some flowers; then the police sent several computerised letters which commiserated with her.

Dear Sir/Madam,
I understand that you have been the victim of a crime.
I am therefore enclosing literature appertaining to your particular crime ...
Although this letter has been sent to you as a result of you unfortunately becoming a victim of crime the police service understands the importance of crime prevention ...

An enclosed leaflet informed her of the various

services available, because the police 'wishes to do all in its power to help victims of crime by providing a quality service that meets your needs':

CRIME DESK
HELP DESK
INTELLIGENCE DESK
KEY CONTACT FOR VICTIM SUPPORT SERVICES
COMMUNITY SERVICES UNIT

It would be tedious to reproduce the whole leaflet. Suffice it to say that a Crime Desk is 'a single centre which reports and records the incidents of crime over the telephone and permits the opportunity to more accurately assess the right resource to respond effectively'.

In the absence of punishment of the offenders, who were after all caught red-handed, my patient considered that the flowers and the mock-compassionate police leaflets were not merely beside the point, but deeply condescending and even insulting. She wanted action against the two big little bastards, not flowers and a computer's sympathy.

But punishment has its limits. My next patient was a member of the tattooed classes, whose ambition was to leave no inch of his epidermis unimproved by art. He told me how he had gone down with a mate to a pub frequented by students the night before to look for a fight, and how between them they had beaten up four of them. As for his missis, who lived in the flat below his, she was winding him up by seeing another bloke, and was looking for a smack in the teef. She deserved it, because she had once given him a smack in the mouf.

'Where are you going now?' I asked him as he left.

'I'm going to get my eye pierced.'

I shrank in horror, but he explained that it was his eyebrow that he meant. He wanted a ring through it.

'I've already done my nipples myself,' he added by way of explanation.

55

I once read a book by a philosopher in which it was maintained that there was no drug yet in existence so powerful in its addictive properties that it could be said truly to remove the ability of a man to act in accordance with his own will. Thus, addiction was essentially a moral problem after all, despite the attempts by social workers, psychiatrists and other verminous do-gooders to persuade us otherwise.

There is, however, one thing known to me which is so utterly addictive that it confounds all human attempts to counteract its effects. I refer, of course, to the payment of Sickness Benefit, the very life-blood (to change the metaphor slightly) of hypochondriasis. How many invalids has it created, how many new and incurable illnesses has it spawned! The arrival of smallpox in the New World was scarcely more devastating in its effect on the health of the population. The British have as little resistance to the Sickness Benefit sickness as the Indians to smallpox, and the only effective vaccine against it so far discovered is self-employment.

Last week, one of my chronics announced as he came through the door that he was 'covered in arthritis'. That was why he had to spend so much on paracetamols. It was a scandal that sufferers such as he should have to pay, when he could name twenty scroungers in his road alone who received more benefits than he, and they weren't even ill.

'Do you know S— Street?' he continued rhetorically. 'Well, it's right next to the hospital, and there's no buses what go down there anyhow. But I know a woman what lives down there called Milly what claims bus fare off the Social every time she goes down the hospital.'

Ah, what wonderful informers and petty spies for a

dictatorship the British would make! They'd deliver up their neighbours to the torture chambers of the secret police just for the pleasure of it, let alone for payment.

One of my patient's symptoms of chronic infirmity was his insatiable need for sex.

'I even have to go down the Golden Eagle and wait for hours till Maggie comes out. She's a bit simple and she'll do it for almost nothing, a couple of fags, like. Mind you, I once nearly got into trouble. There was a notice in the pub which said if you needed sex you could call Gladys, so I did. I was young then and desperate for sex – like I am now. Gladys told me to meet her somewhere and I went, but when I arrived Gladys was working for the CID and they took me down the station. They let me off with a warning, though.'

Suddenly he grew anxious.

'You don't think I'm a finger-ache kind of person, do you, doctor?'

'What's that?'

'Someone who won't work just because he's got an ache in his finger.'

'Oh, no,' I said.

'Because I don't consider myself a fraud. I just can't control my nerves, that's all. I wanted to be like my father and go to work every day. I doted myself on him.'

'Yes,' I said. 'I'm sure.'

A frown passed over his face like a cloud over the sun.

'But if the Social ask me to have a medical to see if I can work, I'm not having one. I'll take a hammer and some petrol with me.'

I smiled as I thought of him hammering his petrol alight.

'I'm serious, doctor, I'd really do it.' He got up to leave. 'Can I have a sick note, please?'

'Of course.'

But what to put in the space for *Reason for absence from work?*
Satyriasis?

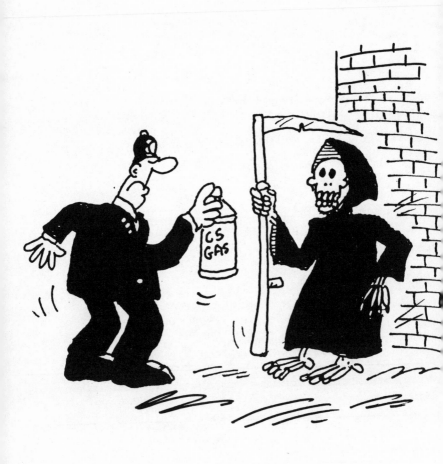

56

According to the late Sir Karl Popper, one could never prove that one's scientific theories were correct, only that, for the moment, they were not incorrect. Obviously, he had never met prisoner Williams.

My hypothesis, recorded in the prison medical notes some three years back when first I came across Williams, was that he would be back in prison very shortly after his release. Here is what I so prophetically wrote:

> Williams says he is a burglar because he needs the money. Since it is unlikely that his economic prospects will have improved since his last spell of freedom, his next spell of freedom will probably also be brief.

Sure enough, here was Williams again, asking for the same sleeping tablets because of his inability to sleep – 'It's my main problem, doctor' – though I must admit he looked a little older, and he thought so too.

'Me 'air's fallen out, doctor, with the worry.'

He was also minus a few teeth, though I failed to enquire as to whether they fell or were pushed.

'How long did you manage to stay on the out this time?' I asked.

'Seven days.'

'And what are you charged with?'

'Two attempteds, one going equipped and two Section 18s.'

The attempteds, perhaps I should explain, were attempted burglaries, while the going equipped entailed apprehension before he even got as far as the attempting.

'Not bad for seven days,' I said. 'What are you pleading?'

'Guilty on the attempteds and going equipped. Mind you, I never took nothing.'

'But you would have done, if you hadn't been caught.'

'Oh yeah, of course.'

'And the Section 18s?'

'Not guilty,' he said, in a tone of injured innocence. 'They was only Section 47s. If they was only trying to pin 47s on me, I'd go guilty.'

An explanation for the uninitiated in the technicalities of the law of assault as laid down in the Offences Against the Persons Act of 1861: the former (GBH) is very much more serious an offence than the latter (ABH), and carries a stiff sentence.

'I only slapped them about a bit. She wasn't even injured, except for a small cut.'

'Who?'

'Me missis. When I came out of prison she introduced me to this bloke, and I shook his hand and had a drink with him in the pub, but then I discovered that she was messing about with him, like. Everyone was laughing at me, so I asked her about it.'

'What happened?'

'She was giving me Miss Cocky, so I gave her a smack on the mouth.'

I tried to get him to see the problem from her point of view: a burglar who spent most of his life in prison was not much of a husband.

'She used to help me on the burglaries, but I always took the rap for her. Last time, I took four TICs off the police if they'd let her go.'

Taken into Considerations (TICs) are the means, roughly speaking, by which known criminals admit to offences they didn't do, in order for the police to clear up crimes they can't solve. As for the police's contention that his assault had been a serious one, it was laughable.

154

'I even went with her to the 'ospital.'

'She had to go to hospital, then?'

'She had a black eye. They kept her in overnight but discharged her first thing next morning. The police are saying it was concussion.'

57

My readers – if I have any – will be pleased to hear that the infantilisation of the British public proceeds apace (I hesitate to add, according to plan).

I was sitting in out-patients last week waiting (in vain, as it transpired) for the arrival of Mr B who had a three o'clock appointment with me. Mr B had been fulsome, indeed obsequious, in his praise of the care he had received while an in-patient, and his thanks had stuck to me as tenaciously and made me feel as unclean as the spittle of a score of drunks in casualty.

It was while I was waiting for him that Sister – who these days is probably called the Manager of something or another – delivered to me a short circular from someone further up the hierarchy of madness. It concerned the recent appointment of DNA Registry Officers.

Now DNA in this context has nothing to do with deoxyribonucleic acid, the manipulation of whose double helix will one day, in the words of a Nigerian witchdoctor with reference to infertility among women, make the impossible to be possible. No, DNA with regard to out-patients means Did Not Attend: the Mr Bs of this world, of whom there are many.

The task of the DNA Registry Officers will be to call up out-patients the evening before their appointment to ask them whether they mean to keep them. The purpose of this, said the circular, is 'to decide about the planning of the care of those who do not intend to attend'.

Plan their care! Plan their punishment would be more like it! I should be all in favour of DNA Registry Officers – the more the better, nearly a third of patients don't turn up, after all – if we were to send in the Hospital Security boys afterwards, to drag defaulters by force from their homes to the entrance of the hospital. There, for a first offence, they would undergo public degradation: for example, they would have their social security or child benefit books ceremonially torn up in front of them by angry, purple-faced consultants.

For second offences, they would be placed in the stocks and pelted with National Health sandwiches (especially sardine), propelled by righteous patients who had arrived on time for their appointments, and thus had earned the delightful privilege. This would doubtless have the advantage of encouraging punctuality among the ill.

For a third offence, defaulters would be publicly bastinadoed by physiotherapists. A day a week would be set aside for this purpose, and the hospital would improve its finances by selling seats for the show. The only problem, I suspect, would be an insufficiency of such seats, which might lead to some slight public disorder.

But punishment of defaulters was the last thing the hospital management had in mind when it sent this circular round to us. On the contrary: the circular said that the DNA Registry Officers would 'concentrate on' those physicians whose clinics had a DNA rate of more than 25 per cent. That's right, I thought, blame the poor old doctor again for the delinquency of his patients! Was there ever a more flagrant case of blaming the victim?

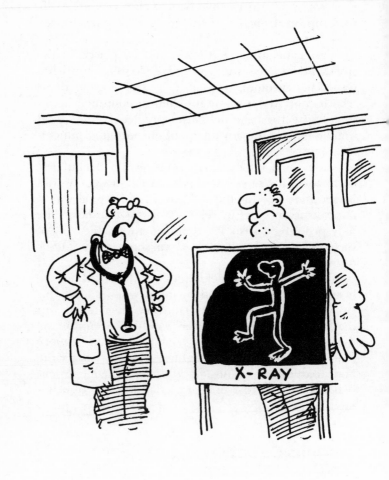

'There's a thin man inside you trying to get out.'

58

I am not exactly an ardent follower of Freud, but there is no doubt that he sometimes had a profound insight into the nature of things, as when he observed that, in his experience, most men were trash. My only objection to this formulation is its mealy-mouthedness: scum would have been more accurate.

Nowhere is this great truth more evident than on Saturday nights in the casualty departments of our general hospitals, to one of which I was called only last weekend. The patient who allegedly required my attention was being held face down on a trolley by two policemen, his arms pinned behind his back and his legs immobilised.

'Good evening,' I said. 'I'm Dr Dalrymple.'

'I'm not answering no questions until you get these fucking pigs off of me.'

I looked at the two policemen, who were wearing surgical gloves in case their *client* (as those who are detained against their will are called these days) had some terrible disease.

'The last time we let him go, doctor, he started to hit the walls. He said there was little green men coming out of them and he was trying to kill them.'

'Little green men,' I repeated.

They were, in fact, about the same colour as the pool of vomitus which was on the floor directly below the client's head.

Now I ask you, is this the company a cultured man such as I should be obliged to keep?

I don't want to be accused of class prejudice, however, so I shall draw my next example from the class to which doctors increasingly belong: that of minor state functionaries.

A young patient of mine, of admittedly modest

intellectual and cultural attainments, decided he wished to leave home and applied to the council (*Working for a better tomorrow*, as the mission statement at the bottom of its stationery puts it) for a flat. His mother, he said, hated him, and had threatened several times that she would kill him one day. This was not an idle threat: she had several convictions for assault.

Public housing being in short supply, it is allocated according to need: need, that is, as estimated by bureaucrats. So when my patient told the housing officer that he had to leave home to avoid being murdered by his mother, the officer agreed it was an emergency. All he required before allocating him a flat, therefore, was confirmation in writing from his mother that she intended to kill him at some time in the near future.

Journalists are just the same. Another patient of mine, a very deserving case, who had worked hard all her life before becoming paralysed from the waist down, was so tired of fruitlessly asking for help from her district council that she called her local newspaper. The gentleman from the fourth estate visited, and asked whether she had been given a date yet.

'A date for what?' my patient asked.

'When you're going to die,' replied the journalist.

'No, I'm paralysed, that's all. They haven't said I'm dying.'

'That's a pity,' said the scribbler. 'Nothing personal, but the readers won't be interested in someone who's only paralysed and isn't dying.'

'I'm sorry, but when I've got a firm date, I'll give you a ring.'

No, ladies and gentlemen, there's no getting away from it: people are trash, to put it mildly.

59

Medical textbooks, even the longest and most pedantic of them, often have curious lacunae. For example, you may search in vain in the index of any of them for a diagnosis which the facts of the case sometimes force upon me, namely that of Cold-hearted Blackguard, which I hope will one day be known to medical science as Dalrymple's Syndrome.

Whether these Blackguards are born or made is a question which is as yet unresolved by even the most sophisticated of research. What is beyond dispute is their existence.

Take last Tuesday. I went into the prison to examine two prisoners on remand for crimes of some magnitude. The first was an attempted murder – and these days you have bloody nearly to succeed to be charged with such a crime, otherwise the charge is reduced to common assault and the matter dropped altogether. Filling in the forms is so tiresome for the police.

'Did you get into trouble at school?' I asked the would-be slayer, as part of my assessment of his character.

'Only the normal theft,' he replied.

'Only the normal theft,' I repeated.

'Yes,' he said, looking at me as if I were being a little slow.

'Tell me,' I asked after a slight pause, 'what is *abnormal* theft?'

'You what?'

'Abnormal theft. What is abnormal theft? If you say that your theft was normal, you must have a conception of what constitutes abnormal theft.'

'I mean I just took a few bicycles,' he said, by now slightly rattled.

Normal: what do we mean by it in fact? There is the

statistician's normal: that is to say, what falls within the range of what 95 per cent of people are or do. Then there is the ideal normal: what we would like people to be or to do. Needless to say, in practice the two normals diverge somewhat.

My second patient was a bugger, both literally and figuratively. Buggery, in fact, was what he was charged with: I didn't know they bothered with legal proceedings these days. But the circumstances were horrific and his wife had pressed charges.

'How,' I asked, 'did you make your wife submit to you?'

'I threatened to kill her,' he said. His tone was entirely matter-of-fact.

'Why did you do that?'

Here I must interrupt my narrative briefly to explain that my patient had been to a counsellor twice a week since his arrest.

'It all goes back to my childhood,' he said.

'How so?' I asked.

'Well, doctor, my father was a drunkard and he used to beat up my mum, so I learned to hate all men.'

I confessed that I didn't see the connection yet.

'Well, doctor. I was 'orrible to my wife so that she would 'ate my father, like my mother 'ated 'im.'

'It couldn't just have been that you were drunk yourself at the time?'

'But it was the weekend, doctor.'

'What has that to do with it?'

'I drank more then, just like my father.'

'Wasn't that because you had a job and you couldn't drink the rest of the week? Just like most people, in fact, including your father and me?'

He looked at me with the malevolence of a spitting cobra.

'I don't need this,' he said, getting up to go.

Sigmund! Thou shouldst be living at this hour:
Felons have need of thee ...

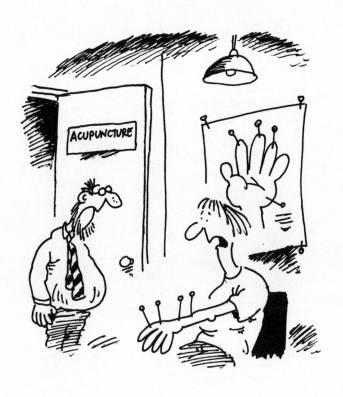

'It's to cure my pins and needles.'

60

Is life worth living? Not in the opinion of one of my patients. He referred to the case of the British murderer recently executed in Georgia.

'That bloke in the electric chair – I would have swapped places with him any time, doctor. He should have tried my life. At least his torture only lasted a few seconds or minutes: mine's lasted for years.'

'Come, come,' I expostulated mildly.

'You don't think I could swap next time they put someone in the electric chair, do you?'

'You mean a kind of international cultural exchange?'

'I'd be better off dead.'

'I don't think such an exchange would be possible.'

'I suppose it's because of the ethics you take.'

For some reason, an image of a tin of Andrews' Liver Salts appeared in my mind's eye.

'If I can't be dead, I'd be better off in a home, doctor.'

'Why?' I asked.

'People in homes don't have to do the washing up. I live with my wife – I don't see what we're gaining by living alone. Sometimes I have these outbursts with her, they get on my nerves, those outbursts, and there comes a time when I start throwing things about the house. I change colour when I get an outburst: it's a purple blotchy kind of feeling, like as if you've got hyperthernia.'

'Oh dear,' I said.

'Yes,' he continued, 'and people in homes don't get no trouble off the neighbours, neither.'

'What trouble?'

'Well, I was going to report them to the police under the Dangerous Dogs Act. Only I didn't because people like them, they don't do nothing at first, but then all of a sudden your windows are broke, and then they bring their dog and make it crap on your path.'

'How do they do that?' I asked.

'Train it, I suppose. You can train a dog to do anything.'

'I don't think so,' I said.

'These irritations may not bother you, doctor, but they bother me. With people like me you don't know how long you can go without an outburst. I should have clinical help. I mean, some people take a shotgun and shoot their neighbours over the hedge.'

'But you wouldn't do anything like that?'

'No. But just because I've got a place of my own doesn't mean I'm going to run it. I've done enough in my life while others have been lying about doing nothing. People don't understand depression – they just say pull yourself together, feed the cat, open the window, and you'll be all right. I want to go in a home.'

'You're a bit young for it,' I said.

'But things get on top of me, like the shopping. Sometimes I feel like getting all the shopping and throwing it around the supermarket.'

'I shouldn't do that,' I said.

'My problem's I'm too timid. If anybody speaks to me I crouch down like a snail. I blame my parents, it's them what made me timid. I even had to go to night school to learn how to speak. When my father took me to the barber he said if you don't behave the barber'll cut your head off. I took him serious.'

'He didn't mean it, I'm sure.'

'Yes, but I didn't know that. Being timid's why I want to kill myself, if I get the chance.'

I looked down at the floor. By my right foot I noticed a little box, put there overnight by the cleaner. It said: 'Rodent bait. Do not touch.'

With a deft movement, I covered it over with a newspaper.